The Male Pelvis

Editor

MUKESH G. HARISINGHANI

MAGNETIC RESONANCE IMAGING CLINICS OF NORTH AMERICA

www.mri.theclinics.com

Consulting Editors
SURESH K. MUKHERJI
LYNNE S. STEINBACH

May 2014 • Volume 22 • Number 2

ELSEVIER

1600 John F. Kennedy Boulevard • Suite 1800 • Philadelphia, Pennsylvania, 19103-2899

http://www.mri.theclinics.com

MRI CLINICS OF NORTH AMERICA Volume 22, Number 2
May 2014 ISSN 1064-9689, ISBN 13: 978-0-323-29713-4

Editor: John Vassallo (j.vassallo@elsevier.com)
Developmental Editor: Yonah Korngold

Magnetic Resonance Imaging Clinics of North America (ISSN 1064-9689) is published quarterly by Elsevier Inc., 360 Park Avenue South, New York, NY 10010-1710. Months of issue are February, May, August, and November. Business and Editorial Offices: 1600 John F. Kennedy Blvd., Ste. 1800, Philadelphia, PA 19103-2899. Customer Service Office: 3251 Riverport Lane, Maryland Heights, MO 63043. Periodicals postage paid at New York, NY and additional mailing offices. Subscription prices are $375.00 per year (domestic individuals), $581.00 per year (domestic institutions), $190.00 per year (domestic students/residents), $420.00 per year (Canadian individuals), $755.00 per year (Canadian institutions), $545.00 per year (international individuals), $755.00 per year (international institutions), and $275.00 per year (international and Canadian students/residents). International air speed delivery is included in all *Clinics* subscription prices. All prices are subject to change without notice. **POSTMASTER:** Send address changes to *Magnetic Resonance Imaging Clinics*, Elsevier Health Sciences Division, Subscription Customer Service, 3251 Riverport Lane, Maryland Heights, MO 63043. Customer Service (orders, claims, online, change of address): Elsevier Health Sciences Division, Subscription Customer Service, 3251 Riverport Lane, Maryland Heights, MO 63043. Tel:1-800-654-2452 (U.S. and Canada); 314-447-8871 (outside U.S. and Canada). Fax: 314-447-8029. E-mail: journalscustomerservice-usa@elsevier.com (for print support); journalsonlinesupport-usa@elsevier.com (for online support).

Reprints. For copies of 100 or more of articles in this publication, please contact the Commercial Reprints Department, Elsevier Inc., 360 Park Avenue South, New York, NY 10010-1710. Tel.: 212-633-3874; Fax: 212-633-3820; E-mail: reprints@elsevier.com.

Magnetic Resonance Imaging Clinics of North America is covered in the *RSNA Index of Imaging Literature*, *MEDLINE/PubMed (Index Medicus)*, and *EMBASE/Excerpta Medica*.

Contributors

CONSULTING EDITORS

SURESH K. MUKHERJI, MD, FACR
Professor and Chairman; W.F. Patenge
Endowed Chair, Department of Radiology,
Michigan State University, East Lansing,
Michigan

LYNNE S. STEINBACH, MD, FACR
Professor of Clinical Radiology and
Orthopaedic Surgery, University of
California-San Francisco, San Francisco,
California

EDITOR

MUKESH G. HARISINGHANI, MD
Professor of Radiology, Harvard Medical
School; Department of Radiology,
Massachusetts General Hospital, Boston,
Massachusetts

AUTHORS

SEYED MAHDI ABTAHI, MD
Division of Abdominal Imaging and
Interventional Radiology, Massachusetts
General Hospital, Boston, Massachusetts

MARIA I. ARGYROPOULOU, MD
Professor, Head of Department, Department
of Clinical Radiology, Medical School,
University of Ioannina, Ioannina, Greece

ANIL S. BHAVSAR, MD
Department of Radiology, University of
Cincinnati Medical Center, Cincinnati, Ohio

LEONARDO K. BITTENCOURT, MD, PhD
Abdominal and Pelvic Imaging, Clinica
de Diagnostico por Imagem (CDPI),
Department of Radiology, Rio de Janeiro
Federal University, Rio de Janeiro, Brazil

JAMES DONOVAN, MD
Department of Urology, University of Cincinnati
Medical Center, Cincinnati, Ohio

AZADEH ELMI, MD
Division of Abdominal Imaging and
Interventional Radiology, Massachusetts
General Hospital, Boston, Massachusetts

ELIZABETH FUREY, MD, FRCPC
Abdominal Imaging, University Health
Network, Mount Sinai and Women's College
Hospital, Toronto, Ontario, Canada

DIMITRIOS GIANNAKIS, MD
Associate Professor, Department of Urology,
Medical School, University of Ioannina,
Ioannina, Greece

ALEXANDER R. GUIMARAES, MD, PhD
Medical Director, Martinos Center for
Biomedical Imaging, Department of
Radiology, Massachusetts General
Hospital, Charlestown, Massachusetts

SUMIT GUPTA, PhD, MRCP
Department of Radiology, University
Hospitals of Leicester NHS Trust, Leicester
General Hospital; University of Leicester,
Glenfield Hospital, Leicester,
United Kingdom

SANDEEP S. HEDGIRE, MD
Division of Abdominal Imaging and
Interventional Radiology, Massachusetts
General Hospital, Boston, Massachusetts

MOIN M. HOOSEIN, MBBS, BSc (Hons), MRCS, FRCR
Consultant Radiologist, Department of Radiology, Leicester General Hospital, University Hospitals of Leicester, Leicester, United Kingdom

KARTIK S. JHAVERI, MD
Abdominal Imaging, University Health Network, Mount Sinai and Women's College Hospital, Toronto, Ontario, Canada

SANJEEVA P. KALVA, MD
Associate Professor; Chief, Division of Interventional Radiology, Department of Radiology, UT Southwestern Medical Center, Dallas, Texas

YUN MAO, MD
Division of Abdominal Imaging and Interventional Radiology, Massachusetts General Hospital, Boston, Massachusetts

ALEXANDRA NTORKOU, MD
Department of Clinical Radiology, University Hospital of Ioannina, Ioannina, Greece

DUANGKAMON PRAPRUTTAM, MD
Division of Abdominal Imaging and Interventional Radiology, Massachusetts General Hospital, Boston, Massachusetts

ARUMUGAM RAJESH, MBBS, FRCR
Consultant Radiologist, Department of Radiology, Leicester General Hospital, University Hospitals of Leicester, Leicester, United Kingdom

RAHUL A. SHETH, MD
Department of Radiology, Massachusetts General Hospital, Boston, Massachusetts

NIKOLAOS SOFIKITIS, MD
Professor, Head of Department, Department of Urology, Medical School, University of Ioannina, Ioannina, Greece

PATRICK D. SUTPHIN, MD, PhD
Assistant Professor, Division of Interventional Radiology, Department of Radiology, UT Southwestern Medical Center, Dallas, Texas

ANASTASIOS SYLAKOS, MD
Department of Urology, Medical School, University of Ioannina, Ioannina, Greece

ATHINA C. TSILI, MD
Lecturer, Department of Clinical Radiology, Medical School, University of Ioannina, Ioannina, Greece

SADHNA VERMA, MD
Associate Professor, Department of Radiology, University of Cincinnati Medical Center, Cincinnati, Ohio

Contents

> MR imaging is the modality of choice for accurate local staging of bladder cancer. In addition, bladder MR imaging helps detect lymph node involvement, and in conjunction with computed tomography, provides complete staging. Familiarity with optimal imaging protocols, normal urinary bladder anatomy, and pathologic MR imaging appearances is essential for the radiologist. Evolving techniques, such as use of diffusion-weighted imaging and lymphotropic nanoparticle-enhanced MR imaging, may further enhance the ability of MR imaging in local and nodal staging.

> Nearly all prostate biopsies are performed via the transrectal ultrasound (TRUS)-guided technique which suffers from its inability to accurately visualize and target suspicious lesions. Advances in prostate MR imaging now allow for the detection of suspicious regions of the prostate gland, opening the door for lesion-directed biopsy techniques. The ability to obtain a definitive histologic grade has become increasingly important due to the rise of active surveillance as a popular method to approach low-grade cancer. Biopsies obtained with MR guidance or MR imaging/transrectal ultrasound fusion can accurately identify and characterize cancers and thus appropriately stratify patients for specific therapies.

> Diffusion-weighted (DW) imaging is playing an increasingly important role in disease detection, prognostication, and monitoring of treatment response. Particularly in the realm of oncology, the potential applications for DW imaging continue to expand. In this article, the authors detail the role of DW imaging for pathologic processes involving the male pelvis. The authors describe the current data, new insights, and ongoing controversies regarding DW imaging of the male pelvis with a particular emphasis on oncologic applications. The authors also discuss imaging techniques and common pitfalls for DW imaging in this anatomic region.

> MR imaging plays a key role in staging evaluation of rectal cancer. The cornerstone of staging MR involves high-resolution T2 imaging orthogonal to the rectal lumen.

The goals of MR staging are identification of patients who will benefit from neoadjuvant therapy prior to surgery to minimize postoperative recurrence and planning of optimal surgical approach. MR provides excellent anatomic visualization of the rectum and mesorectal fascia, allowing for accurate prediction of circumferential resection margin status and tumor stage. MR has an evolving role for the evaluation of neoadjuvant treatment response, further triaging optimal patient treatment and surgical approach.

Penile cancer, although rare in the developed world, has devastating physical and psychological consequences for the patient. Accurate local staging of primary penile cancer can be achieved with magnetic resonance (MR) imaging. This article reviews the normal penile anatomy and MR imaging techniques and features of primary and metastatic penile cancer. Recent advances in penile cancer imaging are discussed.

Magnetic resonance (MR) imaging offers a noninvasive tool for diagnosis of primary and metastatic pelvic tumors. The diagnosis of a pelvic metastatic lesion implies an adverse prognosis and dictates the management strategies. Knowledge of normal MR imaging anatomy of the pelvis and the signal characteristics of normal and abnormal structures is essential for accurate interpretation of pelvic MR imaging. This article reviews imaging manifestations of nodal, visceral, and musculoskeletal metastatic lesions of the pelvis along with current and evolving MR imaging techniques.

Magnetic resonance (MR) imaging of the scrotum has been used as a valuable supplemental diagnostic modality in evaluating scrotal diseases, mostly recommended in cases of inconclusive sonographic findings. Because of the advantages of the technique, MR imaging of the scrotum may provide valuable information in the detection and characterization of various scrotal diseases. The technique may accurately differentiate intratesticular from extratesticular mass lesions and provide important information in the preoperative characterization of the histologic nature of scrotal masses. An accurate estimation of the local extent of testicular carcinomas in patients for whom testis-sparing surgery is planned is possible.

MR angiography is a powerful tool in evaluating anatomy and pathology when applied to the male pelvis. MR angiography produces high-quality images of the arterial system approaching the resolution of CT angiography, without ionizing radiation. Additional advantages include the ability to obtain angiographic images in the absence of contrast material with non–contrast-enhanced MR angiographic techniques. Blood pool contrast agents, such as gadofosveset, have significantly improved the quality of venous system imaging. Steady state imaging with blood pool contrast agents allows for acquisition of superior-quality high-resolution images and other time-intensive techniques.

MAGNETIC RESONANCE IMAGING CLINICS OF NORTH AMERICA

FORTHCOMING ISSUES

August 2014
Hepatobiliary Imaging
Peter S. Liu and Richard G. Abramson, *Editors*

November 2014
MRI of the Knee
Kirkland W. Davis, *Editor*

February 2015
Cardiac MR
Karen Ordovas, *Editor*

RECENT ISSUES

February 2014
Bowel Imaging
Jordi Rimola, *Editor*

November 2013
Imaging of the Pediatric Abdomen and Pelvis
Jonathan R. Dillman and Ethan A. Smith, *Editors*

August 2013
Breast Imaging
Bonnie N. Joe, *Editor*

RELATED INTEREST

Radiologic Clinics of North America, November 2013
Female Pelvic Imaging
Neeraj Lalwani and Theodore J. Dubinsky, *Editors*

PROGRAM OBJECTIVE

The goal of *Magnetic Resonance Imaging Clinics of North America* is to keep practicing physicians up to date with current clinical practice by providing timely articles reviewing the state of the art in patient care.

TARGET AUDIENCE

All practicing physicians and healthcare professionals who provide patient care utilizing findings from Magnetic Resonance Imaging.

LEARNING OBJECTIVES

Upon completion of this activity, participants will be able to:
1. Discuss magnetic resonance imaging of the scrotum, urinary bladder, as well as rectal and penile cancer.
2. Explain male pelvic magnetic resonance angiography.
3. Review magnetic resonance imaging guided prostate biopsy techniques.

ACCREDITATION

The Elsevier Office of Continuing Medical Education (EOCME) is accredited by the Accreditation Council for Continuing Medical Education (ACCME) to provide continuing medical education for physicians.

The EOCME designates this enduring material for a maximum of 15 *AMA PRA Category 1 Credit*(s)™. Physicians should claim only the credit commensurate with the extent of their participation in the activity.

All other health care professionals requesting continuing education credit for this enduring material will be issued a certificate of participation.

DISCLOSURE OF CONFLICTS OF INTEREST

The EOCME assesses conflict of interest with its instructors, faculty, planners, and other individuals who are in a position to control the content of CME activities. All relevant conflicts of interest that are identified are thoroughly vetted by EOCME for fair balance, scientific objectivity, and patient care recommendations. EOCME is committed to providing its learners with CME activities that promote improvements or quality in healthcare and not a specific proprietary business or a commercial interest.

The planning committee, staff, authors and editors listed below have identified no financial relationships or relationships to products or devices they or their spouse/life partner have with commercial interest related to the content of this CME activity:

Seyed Mahdi Abtahi, MD; Maria I. Argyropoulou, MD; Anil S. Bhavsar, MD; Leonardo K. Bittencourt, MD; James Donovan, MD; Azadeh Elmi, MD; Elizabeth Furey, MD, FRCPC; Dimitrios Giannakis, MD; Alexander R. Guimaraes, MD, PhD; Sumit Gupta, PhD, MRCP; Mukesh G. Harisinghani, MD; Sandeep S. Hedgire, MD; Kristen Helm; Moin M. Hoosein, MBBS, BSc (Hons), MRCS, FRCR; Brynne Hunter; Kartik S. Jhaveri, MD; Yun Mao, MD; Jill McNair; Suresh K. Mukherji, MD, FACR; Alexandra Ntorkou, MD; Duangkamon Prapruttam, MD; Arumugam Rajesh, MBBS, FRCR; Rahul A. Sheth, MD; Nikolaos Sofikitis, MD; Lynne S. Steinbach, MD, FACR; Karthikeyan Subramaniam; Patrick D. Sutphin, MD, PhD; Anastasios Sylakos, MD; Athina C. Tsili, MD; John Vassallo; Sadhna Verma, MD.

The planning committee, staff, authors and editors listed below have identified financial relationships or relationships to products or devices they or their spouse/life partner have with commercial interest related to the content of this CME activity:

Sanjeeva P. Kalva, MD has royalties/patents with Amirsys, Inc. and Elsevier, and is a consultant/advisor for Celonova Biosciences, Inc.

UNAPPROVED/OFF-LABEL USE DISCLOSURE

The EOCME requires CME faculty to disclose to the participants:
1. When products or procedures being discussed are off-label, unlabelled, experimental, and/or investigational (not US Food and Drug Administration (FDA) approved); and
2. Any limitations on the information presented, such as data that are preliminary or that represent ongoing research, interim analyses, and/or unsupported opinions. Faculty may discuss information about pharmaceutical agents that is outside of FDA-approved labelling. This information is intended solely for CME and is not intended to promote off-label use of these medications. If you have any questions, contact the medical affairs department of the manufacturer for the most recent prescribing information.

TO ENROLL

To enroll in the *Magnetic Resonance Imaging Clinics of North* Continuing Medical Education program, call customer service at 1-800-654-2452 or sign up online at http://www.theclinics.com/home/cme. The CME program is available to subscribers for an additional annual fee of $250 USD.

METHOD OF PARTICIPATION

In order to claim credit, participants must complete the following:
1. Complete enrolment as indicated above.
2. Read the activity.
3. Complete the CME Test and Evaluation. Participants must achieve a score of 70% on the test. All CME Tests and Evaluations must be completed online.

CME INQUIRIES/SPECIAL NEEDS

For all CME inquiries or special needs, please contact elsevierCME@elsevier.com.

Preface
The Male Pelvis

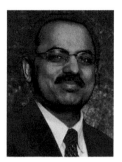

Mukesh G. Harisinghani, MD
Editor

Recent advances in MR imaging have made it the primary modality for evaluating diseases of the male pelvis. These advances include improved coil design, faster imaging techniques, and quantitative assessment tools such as DCE-MR and DWI. Owing to these new improvements, MR has now become the primary modality for evaluating the prostate and rectum with increasing use seen in the clinical assessment of diseases affecting the urinary bladder, penis, scrotum, pelvic vasculature, and lymph nodes. Despite all the advances, care must be taken to ensure the use of optimal imaging technique and protocols to answer the clinical question at hand as the inherent advantage of MR can be negated by poor choice of technique and protocols.

The aim of this issue on "The Male Pelvis" is to provide readers with an overview of current MR imaging as it is applicable to diseases affecting the male pelvis. The sections highlight MR appearances of diseases affecting the male pelvis and also cover technical considerations. The authors have done an exemplary job by contributing excellent and up-to-date articles.

Mukesh G. Harisinghani, MD
Department of Radiology
Massachusetts General Hospital
Harvard Medical School
55 Fruit Street
Boston, MA 02114, USA

E-mail address:
mharisinghani@partners.org

1064-9689/14/$ – see front matter Published by Elsevier Inc.

Magn Reson Imaging Clin N Am 22 (2014) xi
http://dx.doi.org/10.1016/j.mric.2014.02.001
1064-9689/14/$ – see front matter Published by Elsevier Inc.

Erratum

In the November 2013 issue (Volume 21, number 4), in the article "Magnetic Resonance Angiography of the Pediatric Abdomen and Pelvis: Techniques and Imaging Findings," the order of the authors was incorrect. The order of authors should be: Sada DM, Vellody R, Liu PS. Dr Peter S. Liu remains the corresponding author. The complete, correct reference is now: Sada DM, Vellody R, Liu PS. Magnetic Resonance Angiography of the Pediatric Abdomen and Pelvis: Techniques and Imaging Findings. Magn Reson Imaging Clin N Am 2013;21(4):843–60.

Magn Reson Imaging Clin N Am 22 (2014) xiii
http://dx.doi.org/10.1016/j.mric.2014.01.009

Magn Reson Imaging Clin N Am 23 (2014) xiii
http://dx.doi.org/10.1016/j.mric.2014.01.003

MR Imaging of the Urinary Bladder

Moin M. Hoosein, MBBS, BSc (Hons), MRCS, FRCR, Arumugam Rajesh, MBBS, FRCR*

KEYWORDS

- Bladder cancer • Magnetic resonance imaging • Bladder imaging • Staging

KEY POINTS

- Bladder cancer continues to cause significant mortality and morbidity worldwide.
- MR imaging is the imaging modality of choice for accurate local staging, which is fundamental in determining further clinical management, particularly for those with T2 or greater disease.
- Novel MR imaging techniques, such as lymphotropic nanoparticle-enhanced MR imaging and the expanded use of diffusion-weighted imaging, may help further in local and nodal staging of disease.

Bladder cancer continues to remain a cause of more than 100,000 deaths annually worldwide. It is estimated that in the United States alone, 72,570 men and women were diagnosed with bladder cancer in 2013, with an estimated annual death rate of 15,210.

Accurate preoperative staging of bladder cancer is of paramount importance in determining the further management pathway. Radiologic and pathologic staging at initial presentation determines this, and prognosis also depends on this initial staging.

Despite involvement of ionizing radiation, computed tomography (CT) has been shown to be a valuable imaging modality in staging bladder cancer. However, MR imaging is more useful in the local staging of bladder cancer because of its inherent soft tissue resolution, soft tissue contrast, and multiplanar capabilities.[1–5] Because of these combined parameters, clear differentiation between bladder wall layers is possible, therefore allowing for more accurate local staging by differentiating muscle invasive from non–muscle invasive disease, and also extramural invasion. These factors all affect further management and prognosis.

BIOLOGY OF BLADDER CARCINOMA

More than 90% of bladder carcinomas are transitional cell carcinomas derived from the urothelium. About 6% to 8% are squamous cell carcinomas, and 2% are adenocarcinomas.[6] Adenocarcinomas may be either of urachal origin or of non-urachal origin; the latter type is generally thought to arise from metaplasia of chronically irritated transitional epithelium.[7] Pathologic grade, which is based on cellular atypia, nuclear abnormalities, and the number of mitotic figures, is of great prognostic importance.

Several etiologic factors are associated with the development of bladder cancer, but in industrialized countries, cigarette smoking is the most important. Specific chemicals have also been identified as causing bladder cancer, as have several occupational exposures to less well-defined agents including aniline dyes.[8] Treatment with cytostatic drugs, especially cyclophosphamide, is associated with increased risk of bladder cancer, as is treatment with radiotherapy for uterine cancer. In developing countries, especially in the Middle East and parts of Africa, infections with members of the genus *Schistosoma* are

Department of Radiology, Leicester General Hospital, University Hospitals of Leicester, Gwendolen Road, Leicester LE5 4PW, UK
* Corresponding author.
E-mail address: arumugam.rajesh@uhl-tr.nhs.uk

Magn Reson Imaging Clin N Am 22 (2014) 129–134
http://dx.doi.org/10.1016/j.mric.2014.01.001
1064-9689/14/$ – see front matter © 2014 Elsevier Inc. All rights reserved.

responsible for a high incidence of bladder cancer, 75% of which are squamous cell carcinomas. Other risk factors for squamous cell carcinomas include long-term catheterization, nonfunctioning bladder (urinary stasis), and urinary tract calculi.[9]

Muscle-invasive bladder tumors are characterized by defects in the p53 and retinoblastoma tumor suppressor genes, whereas non–muscle-invasive bladder tumors are characterized by activating mutations in the HRAS gene and fibroblast growth factor.[10]

ANATOMY OF THE URINARY BLADDER

The urinary bladder is a musculomembranous sac, predominantly extraperitoneal, its size position and relations varying according to the amount of fluid it contains. Peritoneum covers the superior surface, or dome of the bladder. The bladder receives both ureters posterolaterally, whereas inferiorly, the bladder neck is continuous with the urethra. The orifices of the ureters at the uretero-vesical junction are joined by an elevated ridge covered by mucosa (the interureteric ridge). The trigone describes a triangular region on the internal face of the bladder on the inferior wall, marked at its corners by the ureterovesical junction and the urethra.

The bladder is composed of four layers from inside out: (1) the urothelium (mucosa), (2) the lamina propria (submucosa), (3) the muscularis propria, (4) and the serosa (derived from peritoneum). The tunica mucosa is thin and smooth, continuous, above through the ureters with the lining membrane of the renal tubules, and below with that of the urethra. The thickness of the highly vascular lamina propria varies with the degree of distention of the bladder. The muscularis propria, also known as the detrusor, consists of three layers of unstriated muscular fibers: an external, middle, and an internal layer, although radiologically these are not

Table 1	
TNM staging of urinary bladder cancer	
TNM Guidelines for the Staging of Urinary Bladder Cancer	
Descriptor	**Definition**
Tumor	
Tx	Primary tumor cannot be evaluated
T0	No primary tumor
Ta	Noninvasive papillary carcinoma
Tis	Carcinoma in situ
T1	Tumor invades connective tissue under the epithelium (surface layer)
T2	Tumor invades muscle
T2a	Superficial muscle affected (inner half)
T2b	Deep muscle affected (outer half)
T3	Tumor invades perivesical fat
T3a	Tumor is detected microscopically
T3b	Extravesical tumor is visible macroscopically
T4	Tumor invades the prostate gland, uterus, vagina, pelvic wall, or abdominal wall
Node	
Nx	Regional lymph nodes cannot be evaluated
N0	No regional lymph node metastasis
N1	Metastasis in a single lymph node <2 cm in size
N2	Metastasis in a single lymph node >2 cm but <5 cm in size, or multiple lymph nodes <5 cm in size
N3	Metastasis in a lymph node >5 cm in size
Metastasis	
Mx	Distant metastasis cannot be evaluated
M0	No distant metastasis
M1	Distant metastasis

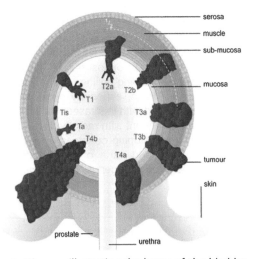

Fig. 1. Diagram illustrating the layers of the bladder wall and tumor staging based on depth of invasion. Also, see **Table 1**.

From Greene FL, Page DL, Fleming ID, et al. Urinary bladder. In: AJCC cancer staging manual. 6th edition. New York: Springer-Verlag; 2002. p. 335–40.

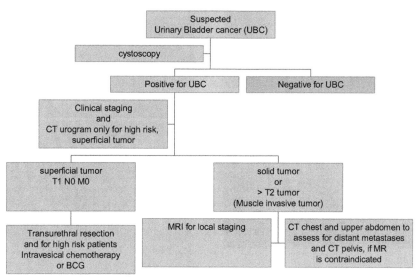

Fig. 2. Algorithm demonstrating the imaging pathway for suspected urinary bladder lesion in our institution. BCG, Bacillus Calmette-Guérin; CT, computed tomography.

differentiated. The serosa invests the superior surface and the upper parts of the lateral surfaces. It is reflected from these onto the abdominal and pelvic walls.

STAGING OF BLADDER CANCER

Staging of bladder cancer is based on the TNM (tumor-node-metastasis) staging system, with T stage representing the degree of bladder wall invasion (Fig. 1, Table 1). Transurethral resection of bladder tumor is often used for T1 disease, whereas partial or total cystectomy or adjuvant therapies are used for stage T2 and beyond, because an adverse side effect of transurethral resection of invasive bladder tumors is local tumor recurrence. Preoperative radiologic distinction between T1 and T2 (or greater) staging of tumors is therefore fundamental to guiding management decisions (Fig. 2).

MR IMAGING TECHNIQUE

The MR imaging protocols used in the figures shown in this article were performed using a Siemens 1.5-T MR imaging scanner (Magnetom Symphony; Siemens Medical Solutions, Erlangen, Germany) (Table 2). A six-channel phased array body coil was used with thin sections and a large matrix. Preliminary localizer sequences are used to evaluate for appropriate coil placement and bladder distention. T1-weighted images (T1WI) are obtained in the axial or coronal plane to give an overview of the pelvis. In particular, the

perivesical fat plane for extravesical involvement, pelvic lymph nodes, and bone metastases can be assessed. On T1WI, urine has low signal intensity (SI), bladder wall intermediate SI, and perivesical fat a high SI. T2-weighted images (T2WI) are obtained in all three orthogonal planes to demonstrate the detrusor muscle well. The detrusor muscle is depicted as a T2 hypointense line and is interrupted in the case of muscle-invasive tumors. Urine has a high SI on T2WI.

Optimal bladder distention is of fundamental importance for accurate diagnosis. Overdistention can result in flat or plaquelike lesions being missed, and underdistention can result in smaller lesions being missed because of detrusor muscle thickening. Some centers advocate use of antiperistaltic agents to prevent artifact from bowel peristalsis; however, we do not routinely use them.

The use of dynamic gadolinium-enhanced sequences as part of a standard protocol varies

Table 2
MR imaging protocol for bladder cancer: adequate patient positioning

MR Imaging Acquisition Parameters[a]	TR	TE	FOV
T2 sagittal	230	100	230
T2 coronal	4700	107	160
T1 axial	499	12	400
T2 axial	2600	100	200

[a] MR imaging acquisition parameters at our institute.

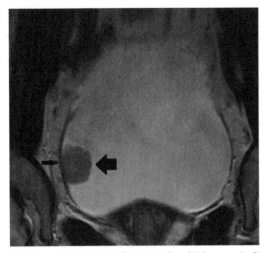

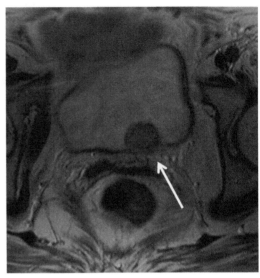

Fig. 3. T2-weighted axial image. The *thick arrow* indicates the tumor. The low signal (*thin arrow*) of the detrusor muscle is uninterrupted in keeping with T1 stage.

Fig. 4. T2-weighted axial image. There is interruption of low signal muscular wall of the bladder (*arrow*) in keeping with T2 tumor.

between institutions. Some studies advocate its use, whereas others have shown no significant advantage.[3,11,12,13]

MR IMAGING STAGING
T Staging

The most important role of MR imaging in bladder cancer in terms of clinical management is to determine the presence of muscle invasion. T1 disease does not involve the detrusor muscle (**Fig. 3**). Conversely, depth of mural invasion can also be assessed and subdivided on MR imaging into T2a and T2b disease (**Fig. 4**). T2WI can

demonstrate macroscopic perivesical spread, seen as a direct extension of the lesion into the perivesical fat tissue and indicating T3b disease (**Fig. 5**). It is important to interpret this in the clinical context, however, because postcystoscopic biopsy imaging can lead to perivesical stranding, which should not be interpreted as disease extension. Such imaging should be delayed until about 4 to 6 weeks postintervention. Conversely, microscopic perivesical spread indicating T3a disease cannot readily be appreciated on CT or MR imaging. Although T1 lesions can be differentiated from T2 lesions or higher with the use of

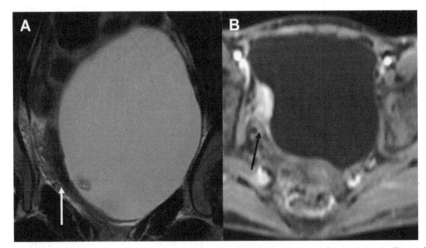

Fig. 5. T2-weighted (*A*) and T1 fat saturated postcontrast (*B*) axial images. The *arrows* indicate bladder wall invasion and perivesicle extension in keeping with a T3b tumor.

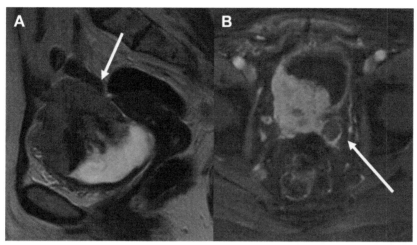

Fig. 6. T2-weighted (*A*) and T1 FS postcontrast (*B*) axial images. The *arrows* indicate small bowel involvement in keeping with T4a tumor.

contrast enhancement, the need for this is usually precluded by histologic confirmation. Invasion of local structures indicating T4 disease is usually well appreciated on MR imaging (**Figs. 6–8**). The overall sensitivity of detecting and staging the primary tumor ranges from 62% to 87.5%.[11,12]

N Staging

The inherent challenge faced with recognition of nodal disease is that it is primarily based on size criteria. Large nodes can be hyperplastic and reactive, and malignant nodes are not always enlarged. These lead to false-positive and false-negative results. Bladder cancer spreads to the paravesical, lateral sacral and presacral nodes, then to the obturator, hypogastric, external iliac and common iliac nodes. Obturator nodes are

involved in 75% of those with nodal disease.[14] The overall sensitivity of detecting nodal metastases based on node size ranges from 64% to 92%.[13,15]

DEVELOPING MR IMAGING TECHNIQUES

The role of diffusion-weighted imaging (DWI) is still being established. DWI can be beneficial in the differentiation of benign and malignant bladder lesions, and of high- and low-grade urinary carcinomas, using quantitative apparent diffusion coefficient measurements. DWI has also been evaluated in terms of staging and efficacy of induction chemotherapy.[16–19] Ultrasmall superparamagnetic iron-oxide–enhanced MR imaging has been reported to improved lymph node staging in several studies, and in patients with bladder and/or prostate cancer, a diagnostic accuracy of

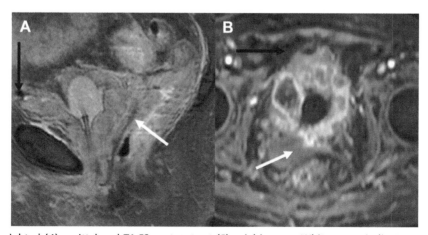

Fig. 7. T2-weighted (*A*) sagittal and T1 FS postcontrast (*B*) axial images. *White arrow* indicates rectal invasion, *black arrow* indicates abdominal wall invasion, both in keeping with stage T4b.

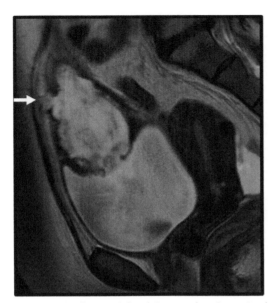

Fig. 8. Sagittal T2-weighted image showing mixed signal intensity mass in the dome extending into the urachal remnant and anterior abdominal wall (*arrow*).

up to 90% has been achieved for detecting metastatic lymph nodes.[20]

SUMMARY

MR imaging is the modality of choice for accurate local staging of bladder cancer. In addition, bladder MR imaging helps detect lymph node involvement, and in conjunction with CT, provides complete staging. Familiarity with optimal imaging protocols, normal urinary bladder anatomy, and pathologic MR imaging appearances is essential for the radiologist. Evolving techniques, such as use of DWI and lymphotropic nanoparticle-enhanced MR imaging, may further enhance the ability of MR imaging in local and nodal staging.

REFERENCES

1. Beyersdorff D, Zhang J, Schöder H, et al. Bladder cancer: can imaging change patient management? Curr Opin Urol 2008;18(1):98–104.
2. Kirkali Z, Chan T, Manoharan M, et al. Bladder cancer: epidemiology, staging and grading, and diagnosis. Urology 2005;66(6 Suppl 1):4–34.
3. Rajesh A, Sokhi HK, Fung R, et al. Bladder cancer: evaluation of staging accuracy using dynamic MRI. Clin Radiol 2011;66(12):1140–5.
4. Blake MA, Kalra MK. Imaging of urinary tract tumors. Cancer Treat Res 2008;143:299–317.
5. Setty BN, Holalkere NS, Sahani DV, et al. State-of-the-art cross-sectional imaging in bladder cancer. Curr Probl Diagn Radiol 2007;36(2):83–96.
6. Mostofi FK, Davis CJ, Sesterhenn IA. Pathology of tumors of the urinary tract. In: Skinner DG, Lieskovsky G, editors. Diagnosis and management of genitourinary cancer. Philadelphia: WB Saunders; 1988. p. 83–117.
7. Wilson TG, Pritchett TR, Lieskovsky G, et al. Primary adenocarcinoma of bladder. Urology 1991;38(3): 223–6.
8. Cohen SM, Johansson SL. Epidemiology and etiology of bladder cancer. Urol Clin North Am 1992; 19(3):421–8.
9. Johansson SL, Cohen SM. Epidemiology and etiology of bladder cancer. Semin Surg Oncol 1997; 13(5):291–8.
10. Wu XR. Urothelial tumorigenesis: a tale of divergent pathways. Nat Rev Cancer 2005;5(9):713–25.
11. Kim B, Semelka RC, Ascher SM, et al. Bladder tumor staging: comparison of contrast-enhanced CT, T1- and T2-weighted MR imaging, dynamic gadolinium-enhanced imaging, and late gadolinium-enhanced imaging. Radiology 1994;193(1):239–45.
12. Tekes A, Kamel I, Imam K, et al. Dynamic MRI of bladder cancer: evaluation of staging accuracy. AJR Am J Roentgenol 2005;184(1):121–7.
13. Daneshmand S, Ahmadi H, Huynh LN, et al. Preoperative staging of invasive bladder cancer with dynamic gadolinium-enhanced magnetic resonance imaging: results from a prospective study. Urology 2012;80(6):1313–8.
14. Husband JE. CT/MRI of nodal metastases in pelvic cancer. Canc Imag 2002;2:123–9.
15. Paik ML, Scolieri MJ, Brown SL, et al. Limitations of computerized tomography in staging invasive bladder cancer before radical cystectomy. J Urol 2000;163(6):1693–6.
16. Watanabe H, Kanematsu M, Kondo H, et al. Preoperative T staging of urinary bladder cancer: does diffusion-weighted MRI have supplementary value? AJR Am J Roentgenol 2009;192(5):1361–6.
17. Avcu S, Koseoglu MN, Ceylan K, et al. The value of diffusion-weighted MRI in the diagnosis of malignant and benign urinary bladder lesions. Br J Radiol 2011;84(1006):875–82.
18. Takeuchi M, Sasaki S, Ito M, et al. Urinary bladder cancer: diffusion-weighted MR imaging–accuracy for diagnosing T stage and estimating histologic grade. Radiology 2009;251(1):112–21.
19. Verma S, Rajesh A, Prasad SR, et al. Urinary bladder cancer: role of MR imaging. Radiographics 2012; 32(2):371–87.
20. Thoeny HC, Triantafyllou M, Birkhaeuser FD, et al. Combined ultrasmall superparamagnetic particles of iron oxide-enhanced and diffusion-weighted magnetic resonance imaging reliably detect pelvic lymph node metastases in normal-sized nodes of bladder and prostate cancer patients. Eur Urol 2009;55(4):761–9.

MR Imaging–Guided Prostate Biopsy Techniques

Sadhna Verma, MD[a],*, Anil S. Bhavsar, MD[a],
James Donovan, MD[b]

KEYWORDS

- Prostate cancer • MR imaging • Diagnostic • Transrectal ultrasound–guided biopsy
- MR imaging/ultrasound fusion • MR imaging–guided prostate biopsy

KEY POINTS

- A diagnosis of localized prostate cancer has always represented a clinical challenge.
- Nearly all prostate biopsies are performed via the transrectal ultrasound-guided (TRUS) technique, which suffers from multiple limitations owing to its inability to accurately visualize and target suspicious lesions.
- Advances in prostate MR imaging now allow for direct visualization of suspicious regions of the prostate gland, opening the door for lesion-directed biopsy techniques.
- Advancing biopsy techniques include direct MR imaging guidance and MR imaging/ultrasound fusion.

INTRODUCTION

Prostate cancer is the second most frequently diagnosed cancer worldwide and the sixth leading cause of cancer death in men, accounting for 14% of total new cancer cases and 6% of total cancer deaths.[1] Fortunately, it is now estimated that 92% of new cases of prostate cancer are clinically localized at diagnosis, for which the 5-year relative survival approaches 100%.[2] Unfortunately, current state-of-the-art diagnostic and staging algorithms that are based on TRUS biopsies have substantial limitations resulting in unnecessary biopsies, inaccurate characterization of prostate cancer aggressiveness, patient anxiety, morbidity, and increased cost. Optimizing treatment strategies requires a careful establishment of an individual's prognosis to avoid unnecessary therapy-induced morbidity or treatment failure. Fundamental to this effort is the ability to achieve a reasonable degree of accuracy for preoperative staging. Initially in this report, current methods and recommendations for prostate screening are discussed. A discussion regarding current paradigms in prostate cancer biopsy ensues.

The two most commonly used tests for diagnosis of prostate cancer are serum prostate-specific antigen (PSA) level measurement and digital rectal examination (DRE).[3] However, current recommendations are evolving given the controversies surrounding the potential benefits and limitations of PSA testing. The American Urological Association (AUA) currently recommends an individualized approach in concert with shared decision making with regards to screening men between 40 and 69 years of age. Individuals who are at high risk (ie, positive family history or African American race) can begin screening at age 40 if both physician and patient agree on the risks and benefits. The same principles apply to patients between 55 and 69 years. The AUA does not currently recommend routine screening of

Disclosures: None.
[a] Department of Radiology, University of Cincinnati Medical Center, 234 Goodman Street, PO Box 670761, Cincinnati, OH 45267–0761, USA; [b] Department of Urology, University of Cincinnati Medical Center, 234 Goodman Street, PO Box 670761, Cincinnati, OH 45267–0761, USA
* Corresponding author.
E-mail address: drsadhnaverma@gmail.com

individuals older than 70 years of age or any man with a less than 10- to 15-year life expectancy.

When prostate cancer is suspected either on the basis of elevated serum PSA levels or abnormal DRE, the diagnosis must be confirmed via biopsy. Prostate biopsies to diagnose or exclude cancer are currently performed approximately 1 million times annually in the United States.[4] Nearly all are performed using the TRUS technique, initially introduced approximately 25 years ago.[5] This technique is performed without knowing the exact tumor location within the prostate (blind biopsy). Currently, prostate cancer is the only major cancer in which diagnosis is routinely made with a blind biopsy of the organ. Unfortunately, microfocal cancers of little clinical significance are frequently detected with blind biopsies.[6] Conversely, for first-time patients, the incidence of false-negative biopsies (ie, serious tumors not detected) may in first-time biopsies be as high as 35%.[7] In addition, the prostate cancer detection rate of TRUS-guided biopsy decreases with every repeat biopsy and increases with the number of cores collected. The increase in detection rate could be attributed to better systematic sampling approach of TRUS biopsies. In comparison, cancer detection rates of targeted biopsy techniques, such as MR imaging or MR imaging/TRUS–directed biopsies, have been shown to be not affected by prior biopsies.[8]

After a diagnosis of low-risk localized prostate cancer (based on clinical stage, PSA, and Gleason grade), approximately 90% of patients elect definitive treatment. This includes either surgery or radiation; the remaining 10% of men choose an active surveillance plan.[9] Active surveillance refers to the close monitoring of patients with favorable-risk prostate cancer by keeping track of serial PSAs, having regular DREs, and undergoing periodic biopsies. Appropriate treatment is provided to active surveillance patients who show evidence of disease progression (either increase tumor volume or increase in Gleason grade). Studies show that prior to initiating patients into active surveillance, a restaging biopsy of the prostate improves selection by excluding up to 30% of those with higher volume or higher stage/grade disease.[10] Thus, accurate disease characterization at diagnosis is paramount.

Multiparametric MR imaging of the prostate is capable of detecting clinically relevant prostate cancer. Although data currently suggest that MR imaging has the potential to assess the biologic aggressiveness of the tumor, it does not replace the need for biopsy histopathologic verification at this time.[11–13] Instead, it is imperative to obtain biopsies of tumor-suspicious areas within the prostate using a combination of TRUS and MR imaging guidance. A recent systematic review showed that the efficiency of the targeted sampling technique is superior to the standard approach of blind biopsies (70% vs 40%).[14]

All MR imaging–guided prostate biopsies begin with a diagnostic prostate MR. According to the European Society of Urogenital Radiology "Prostate MR Guidelines 2012," this includes a combination of a T2-weighted sequence and 2 functional sequences (diffusion-weighted images with either a dynamic contrast-enhanced MR imaging sequence or MR imaging spectroscopy) (Fig. 1).[15]

High-quality diagnostic preprocedural prostate MR imaging is essential for accurate biopsy planning.

METHODS OF MR IMAGING–GUIDED PROSTATE BIOPSY

Three methods of MR imaging guidance are currently available for performance of targeted

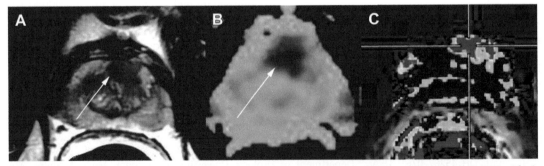

Fig. 1. Multiparametric prostate MR imaging demonstrating an anterior lesion in a 63-year-old patient with rising PSA, 8.6 to 12.5, over 5 years. Two sets of systematic TRUS biopsies were negative. Axial T2-weighted image shows a hypointense left anterior lesion (*A, arrow*) with restricted diffusion on apparent diffusion coefficient map derived from diffusion-weighted imaging (*B, arrow*), and early wash-in/washout on dynamic contrast images (*C*) which is highly suspicious for malignancy. This region was not included in the systematic TRUS biopsy zones.

prostate biopsies cognitive fusion, direct MR imaging–guided biopsy, and software coregistration of a stored MR imaging with real-time ultrasound using a fusion device. Each method has its advantages and disadvantages.

Cognitive Fusion

Cognitive fusion is simple, quick, and requires no additional equipment beyond MR imaging and a conventional TRUS facility. Suspicious areas detected on a prior diagnostic MR imaging are biopsied using TRUS. Because suspicious lesions are localized and detected on MR imaging, targeted biopsy of the corresponding region on TRUS is expected to yield better outcomes than random, blind biopsies of the prostate. Specialized training beyond conventional TRUS biopsy is not required for an ultrasound operator. One recent study suggests that cognitive fusion yields improved accuracy over conventional systematic blind biopsy.[14] A disadvantage of cognitive fusion is the potential for human error in the extrapolation from MR imaging to TRUS without an actual overlay for targeting.

MR Imaging–Guided Prostate Biopsy

The ability to visualize suspicious prostate areas on MR imaging allows for lesion-directed biopsy under MR imaging guidance. This is possible because of the drastically increased speed of MR imaging in the past two decades along with recent advances in computer-based accurate biopsy needle guidance tools. This provides the individual performing the procedure the ability to track the path of the biopsy needle and confirm its position in the lesion of interest prior to performing the biopsy.

MR imaging–guided prostate biopsies have been performed in low-field open MR imaging and the widely available closed-bore MR imaging scanners with 1.5-T or 3-T field strengths.[16–26] The low-field MR imaging allows for easier access to patients, whereas the closed-bore scanner offers a much higher signal-to-noise ratio, allowing for better visualization of the lesion. As for the biopsy approach, a transrectal approach is the preferred method given that it is considered less invasive.[16,17,19–22,24,25]

The MR imaging–guided biopsy is generally performed on a separate date from the diagnostic planning MR imaging. It can follow a same-day diagnostic study if desired. Oral fluoroquinolones are given before and after the biopsy. The actual MR imaging–guided biopsy is performed in bore, or within the MR imaging tube. Patients are generally placed in the prone position. A body phased-array or cardiac coil is placed on the patient's lower back and the MR biopsy device is inserted into the rectum via the endorectal needle guide (**Fig. 2**). Multiplanar localization sequences are performed to identify the regions of interest, typically using a T2-weighted fast spin-echo sequence. The gadolinium-filled needle guide is then directed toward the lesion by means of the prostate biopsy device and guidance sequences are performed between needle guide adjustments. Automated software assists needle placement by providing automated adjustment parameters for the needle (**Fig. 3**). The guidance sequences used are usually T2-weighted fast spin-echo or single-shot fast spin-echo obtained either in the sagittal or oblique axial planes that contain the needle.[20,27,28]

Diagnostic images from the preprocedural prostate MR imaging are fused with contemporaneous MR images to confirm biopsy needle localization. Patients are rescanned to confirm needle localization. Typically, only a few targeted cores are taken. Although most MR imaging–guided biopsies can be completed within 60 to 90 minutes, several factors play a role in longer procedure times. This is largely dependent on the number of biopsies performed and experience of the operator.[19,22] Reported complications include self-limiting hematuria, uncomplicated urinary tract infections, and mild pain.[22] Overall, advantages of this method are the limited number of cores taken,

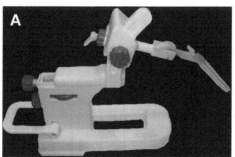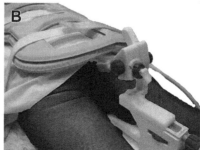

Fig. 2. Biopsy device with needle guide attached (*A*). The needle guide is placed endorectally (*B*).

A   **B**

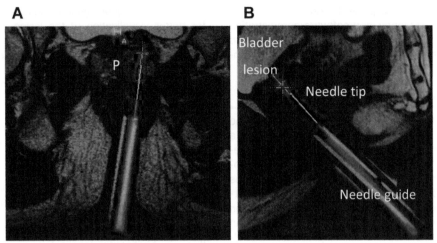

Fig. 3. Direct in-bore MR imaging–guided biopsy of an anterior prostate lesion. The same patient in **Fig. 1** returned for an MR imaging–guided biopsy. After positioning the patient and placing the needle guide in the rectum, a T2-weighted sequence (*A*) is obtained to identify the biopsy target. The needle guide is directed toward the target using a computer-aided technique. After confirming the appropriate position of the needle guide, an 18-gauge MR-compatible biopsy needle is inserted through the guide and biopsy samples are obtained. Additional sagittal T2-weighted images (*B*) were obtained along the axis of the needle guide to confirm the position of the needle in the targeted region. Pathology analysis of the specimens yielded Gleason score 8 adenocarcinoma. P, prostate.

the exact localization of the biopsy, and the reduced detection of insignificant tumors. Disadvantages include the time taken for the biopsies (which includes in-bore time) and the cost expenses for the two MR sessions that are required to obtain the biopsy specimens.[15,29–31]

MR Imaging/Ultrasound Fusion Biopsy

The fusion of MR imaging and TRUS technology offers an alternative to performing targeted prostate biopsies in bore. This technique is performed by coregistering preacquired MR images with

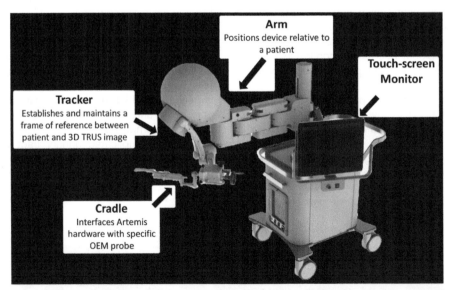

Fig. 4. Artemis fusion device; FDA-approved commercial model. When the TRUS probe is rotated (the tracking arm is stabilized and held stationary during the rotation), encoders in the tracking mechanism transmit orientation and position of the transducer tip to software that displays and records location on the monitor. During the scan, 2-D images are digitized and reconstructed into a 3-D image. A model of the prostate is generated from the 3-D image. MR imaging fusion, biopsy, and tracking of biopsy sites can be performed on the reconstructed prostate model. (*Courtesy of* Eigen, Grass Valley, CA.)

real-time TRUS and has shown its value in improving the quality of prostate biopsies by targeting regions suspicious for tumor. The primary advantage of MR imaging/TRUS fusion technique is that it does not require MR imaging room time for interventional procedures, saving cost and allowing for quicker turnover. MR imaging/TRUS fusion was first used in central nervous system applications then adapted for use in prostate brachytherapy.[32,33]

MR imaging/TRUS fusion–guided biopsy synergistically combines the strengths of each modality

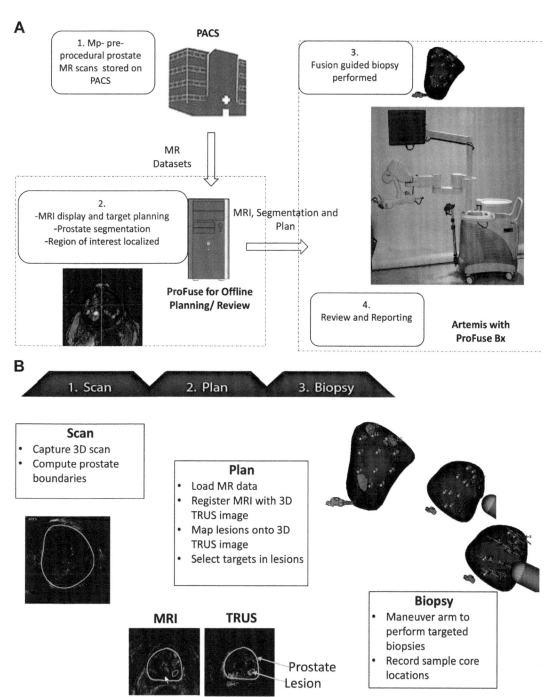

Fig. 5. Fusion workflow, prostate segmentation, and target planning (*A*). Fusion-guided biopsy workflow (*B*). MP, multiparametric; PACS, picture archiving and communication system; ProFuse, multimodality image fusion software (Eigen, Grass Valley, CA, USA). ([*A*] *Courtesy of* Eigen, Grass Valley, CA.)

to overcome the weakness in the other to provide the increased specificity and sensitivity of the MR image with the portability and efficiency of the TRUS system. This combination eliminates the drawbacks of MR imaging–guided biopsy (high costs, long intervention time, and poor ergonomics)[34] while providing the sensitivity and specificity of MR imaging delivered on the US platform in real-time.[15] During an MRI-targeted/US-guided fusion prostate biopsy procedure, biopsies are taken from the MRI areas suspicious for cancer and sampling of standard peripheral zone segments. The value of MR imaging/TRUS prostate biopsy can be appreciated in several different clinical scenarios: (1) detection of anterior prostate cancer which would never be sampled in traditional TRUS prostate biopsies, (2) identification of suspicious targets in large prostates, and (3) in the surveillance of men with low grade prostate cancer managed in "active surveillance" protocols.[30,35–41]

The primary challenge of MR imaging/TRUS fusion–guided procedures is accounting for the deformation of the prostate between the preoperative planning MR imaging acquisition and real-time TRUS-guided biopsy. The prostate can considerably deform during a TRUS intervention due to patient movement and ultrasound probe pressure, especially in the posterior regions of the prostate.[42] Likewise, the same can occur during a prostate MR examination as a result of the endorectal coil. Differences in patient orientation between MR imaging and TRUS (supine vs left lateral decubitus or lithotomy) add to the complexity of the deformation. Two FDA-cleared fusion devices—PercuNav (Philips, Andover, MA, USA) and Real-time virtual sonography (RVS) (Hitachi, Tarrytown, NY, USA)—perform rigid fusion between the preprocedure MR imaging and intraprocedure TRUS volumes.[42,43] The

PercuNav system has undergone the most years of clinical testing.[30] It uses an external magnetic field generator to perform biopsy-site localization and tracking. One study showed that prostate cancer detection highly correlated with degree of suspicion on MR imaging (90% of cases).[44] To assist the rigid fusion of MR imaging and TRUS, Xu and colleagues[43] have recommended the use of an endorectal coil during MR imaging acquisition that simulates the deformation caused by the TRUS probe in addition to boosting image quality. The RVS system also uses magnetic field localization; however, clinical experience with this system is limited.[42,45] Ukimura and colleagues[42] have experimented with MR imaging acquisition using a plastic outer frame shaped like a TRUS probe. This approximates the deformation seen in a TRUS-guided procedure and improves the accuracy of the rigid fusion in the RVS system. Deformable registration algorithms (although more complex than rigid fusion algorithms) may be necessary to compensate for the changes in gland shape during MR imaging acquisition and TRUS-guided procedure. The Urostation device (Koelis, La Tronche, France) uses elastic fusion technology to warp the preprocedure MR imaging and intraprocedure TRUS volumes. Using a semiautomatic morphologic contouring process, a 3-D outline of the prostate is obtained individually for both the MR and TRUS volumes. One of the outlines is then smoothly deformed using elastic registration such that the MR imaging outlines match the TRUS prostate outlines. For targeting, the Urostation uses a retrospective targeting system; that is, the biopsy is taken and then a scan is performed to ensure placement position. It has been suggested that this targeting system is highly accurate. The ability to register actual biopsy trajectory and

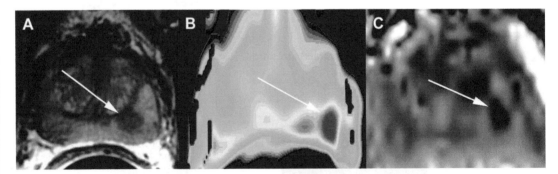

Fig. 6. A 59-year-old man with progressively increasing PSA level for 2 years, reaching 6.42 ng/mL, and 1 prior negative TRUS biopsy. T2-weighted axial MR image demonstrates a nodule in the peripheral zone, midgland level with focal low signal (A, arrow). DCE image shows early wash-in and washout (B, arrow). Diffusion-weighted imaging; axial MR image with an apparent diffusion coefficient value of 0.82 × 10-3 m²/s in the left midgland nodule (C, arrow). This lesion was classified as suspicious for malignancy based on the multiparametric MR imaging features.

perform elastic MR imaging/TRUS fusion should be considered a significant advantage for future focal therapy applications.[46]

The Artemis device (Eigen, Grass Valley, California) is a 3-D ultrasound-guided prostate biopsy system used at the authors' institution (Fig. 4). This device has the ability to plan, record, and prospectively navigate to biopsy targets (eg, systematic 12-core, custom, and revisit biopsy plans).[47] Additionally, in conjunction with proprietary segmentation software, the device allows MR imaging/TRUS fusion–guided biopsies. In a typical workflow (Fig. 5A), multiplanar images from the preprocedural diagnostic MR imaging are uploaded into a segmentation software package. Using this software, a radiologist segments the prostate and marks suspicious areas on the 3-D MR imaging volume. The suspicious regions can be further classified on the degree of suspicion as low, moderate, and high. These data are then electronically transferred to the Artemis device and fused with real-time ultrasound during the procedure (see Fig. 5B). For targeting, the Artemis device incorporates a mechanical arm with encoders that track the arm movement. The arm supports the rectal probe and guides the biopsy needle to targets in the prostate.[48] Initially, the rectal probe is inserted into the patient. Once the probe is in position, it is rotated about its axis to obtain sequential 2-D images that are reconstructed into a 3-D TRUS volume. The device then fuses the 3-D MR imaging and TRUS volumes using deformable surface-based registration of the segmented MR imaging and TRUS surfaces followed by elastic warping.[49] Biopsies of suspicious areas are performed on this fused 3-D model (Figs. 6 and 7).[30]

Technologies to perform image fusion are evolving. Table 1 summarizes the key features of the five devices currently cleared by the Food and Drug Administration.

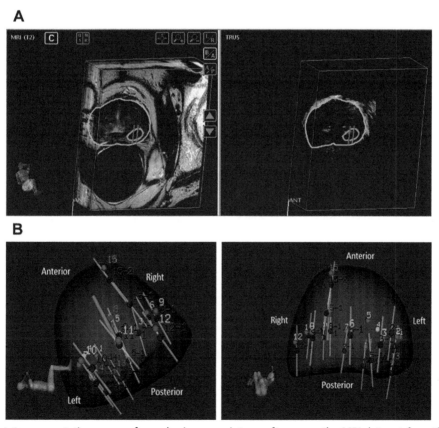

Fig. 7. Prostate segmentation was performed using proprietary software on the MRI data set from the patient in Fig. 6 to produce a 3-D model of the prostate including the target. (A) During biopsy, real-time ultrasound generated a 3-D ultrasound model of the prostate. The two models were then dynamically fused and visualized side-by-side. (B) Systematic and targeted biopsies were obtained, generating a final 3-D model demonstrating the location of all biopsy cores (light brown lines). Targeted biopsies in this patient revealed 2 cores positive for adenocarcinoma (3.5-4 mm; Gleason score 7 = 3 + 4). Further prostatectomy confirmed MR imaging findings.

Table 1
Devices currently approved by the United States Food and Drug Administration for the purpose of MR imaging-TRUS fusion guided prostate biopsy

Manufacturer/ Device	510(k) Clearance Year	Tracking Mechanism	MR imaging/ TRUS Fusion Mechanism
Philips/PercuNav	2005	Prospective targeting, electromagnetic tracking with rigid motion compensation	Rigid
Eigen/Artemis	2008	Prospective targeting, mechanical tracking with rigid motion compensation	Elastic
Koelis/Urostation	2010	Retrospective targeting, real-time TRUS-TRUS elastic registration-based tracking	Elastic
Hitachi/RVS	2010	Prospective targeting, electromagnetic tracking	Rigid
GeoScan Medical Lakewood Ranch, FL, USA/BioJet	2012	Prospective targeting, mechanical arm with encoders; uses stepper	Rigid

SUMMARY

Prostate biopsy is essential for diagnosis and management of prostate cancer. The information obtained from prostate biopsy is increasingly relevant as active surveillance becomes a more common management strategy and focal therapy clinical trials emerge. With active surveillance becoming a popular method to approach low-grade cancers, obtaining an accurate diagnosis of volume and grade is critical to risk stratification and appropriate selection of candidates. Multiparametric MR imaging is currently the best noninvasive imaging modality for diagnosis of prostate cancer, providing some indication of histologic grade. With the benefit of MRI targeting, biopsy results obtained with the fusion devices can accurately identify and characterize cancers and appropriately stratify patients for specific management strategies.

REFERENCES

1. Jemal A, Bray F, Center MM, et al. Global cancer statistics. CA Cancer J Clin 2011;61(2):69–90.
2. Jemal A, Siegel R, Xu J, et al. Cancer statistics. CA Cancer J Clin 2010;60(5):277–300.
3. Thompson I, Thrasher JB, Aus G, et al. Guideline for the management of clinically localized prostate cancer: 2007 update. J Urol 2007;177(6):2106–31.
4. Welch HG, Fisher ES, Gottlieb DJ, et al. Detection of prostate cancer via biopsy in the Medicare-SEER population during the PSA era. J Natl Cancer Inst 2007;99(18):1395–400.
5. Hodge KK, McNeal JE, Stamey TA. Ultrasound guided transrectal core biopsies of the palpably abnormal prostate. J Urol 1989;142(1):66–70.
6. Cooperberg MR, Broering JM, Kantoff PW, et al. Contemporary trends in low risk prostate cancer: risk assessment and treatment. J Urol 2007;178(3 Pt 2):S14–9.
7. Taira AV, Merrick GS, Galbreath RW, et al. Performance of transperineal template-guided mapping biopsy in detecting prostate cancer in the initial and repeat biopsy setting. Prostate Cancer Prostatic Dis 2010;13(1):71–7.
8. Durmus T, Reichelt U, Huppertz A, et al. MRI-guided biopsy of the prostate: correlation between the cancer detection rate and the number of previous negative TRUS biopsies. Diagn Interv Radiol 2013;19:411–7.
9. Cooperberg MR, Broering JM, Carroll PR. Time trends and local variation in primary treatment of localized prostate cancer. J Clin Oncol 2010;28(7):1117–23.
10. Berglund RK, Masterson TA, Vora KC, et al. Pathological upgrading and up staging with immediate repeat biopsy in patients eligible for active surveillance. J Urol 2008;180(5):1964–7 [discussion: 1967–8].
11. Tamada T, Sone T, Jo Y, et al. Apparent diffusion coefficient values in peripheral and transition zones of the prostate: comparison between normal and malignant prostatic tissues and correlation with histologic grade. J Magn Reson Imaging 2008;28(3):720–6.
12. Turkbey B, Shah VP, Pang Y, et al. Is apparent diffusion coefficient associated with clinical risk scores for prostate cancers that are visible on 3-T MR images? Radiology 2011;258(2):488–95.
13. Woodfield CA, Tung GA, Grand DJ, et al. Diffusion-weighted MRI of peripheral zone prostate cancer: comparison of tumor apparent diffusion coefficient with Gleason score and percentage of tumor on core biopsy. AJR Am J Roentgenol 2010;194(4):W316–22.

14. Moore CM, Robertson NL, Arsanious N, et al. Image-guided prostate biopsy using magnetic resonance imaging-derived targets: a systematic review. Eur Urol 2013;63(1):125–40.

15. Barentsz JO, Richenberg J, Clements R, et al. ESUR prostate MR guidelines 2012. Eur Radiol 2012;22(4): 746–57.

16. Anastasiadis AG, Lichy MP, Nagele U, et al. MRI-guided biopsy of the prostate increases diagnostic performance in men with elevated or increasing PSA levels after previous negative TRUS biopsies. Eur Urol 2006;50(4):738–48 [discussion: 748–9].

17. Beyersdorff D, Winkel A, Hamm B, et al. MR imaging-guided prostate biopsy with a closed MR unit at 1.5 T: initial results. Radiology 2005;234(2): 576–81.

18. D'Amico AV, Tempany CM, Cormack R, et al. Transperineal magnetic resonance image guided prostate biopsy. J Urol 2000;164(2):385–7.

19. Engelhard K, Hollenbach HP, Kiefer B, et al. Prostate biopsy in the supine position in a standard 1.5-T scanner under real time MR-imaging control using a MR-compatible endorectal biopsy device. Eur Radiol 2006;16(6):1237–43.

20. Franiel T, Stephan C, Erbersdobler A, et al. Areas suspicious for prostate cancer: MR-guided biopsy in patients with at least one transrectal US-guided biopsy with a negative finding–multiparametric MR imaging for detection and biopsy planning. Radiology 2011;259(1):162–72.

21. Hambrock T, Futterer JJ, Huisman HJ, et al. Thirty-two-channel coil 3T magnetic resonance-guided biopsies of prostate tumor suspicious regions identified on multimodality 3T magnetic resonance imaging: technique and feasibility. Invest Radiol 2008; 43(10):686–94.

22. Hambrock T, Somford DM, Hoeks C, et al. Magnetic resonance imaging guided prostate biopsy in men with repeat negative biopsies and increased prostate specific antigen. J Urol 2010;183(2):520–7.

23. Hata N, Jinzaki M, Kacher D, et al. MR imaging-guided prostate biopsy with surgical navigation software: device validation and feasibility. Radiology 2001;220(1):263–8.

24. Susil RC, Menard C, Krieger A, et al. Transrectal prostate biopsy and fiducial marker placement in a standard 1.5T magnetic resonance imaging scanner. J Urol 2006;175(1):113–20.

25. Yakar D, Hambrock T, Hoeks C, et al. Magnetic resonance-guided biopsy of the prostate: feasibility, technique, and clinical applications. Top Magn Reson Imaging 2008;19(6):291–5.

26. Zangos S, Eichler K, Engelmann K, et al. MR-guided transgluteal biopsies with an open low-field system in patients with clinically suspected prostate cancer: technique and preliminary results. Eur Radiol 2005; 15(1):174–82.

27. Futterer JJ, Verma S, Hambrock T, et al. High-risk prostate cancer: value of multi-modality 3T MRI-guided biopsies after previous negative biopsies. Abdom Imaging 2012;37(5):892–6.

28. Yacoub JH, Verma S, Moulton JS, et al. Imaging-guided prostate biopsy: conventional and emerging techniques. Radiographics 2012;32(3):819–37.

29. Hoeks CM, Schouten MG, Bomers JG, et al. Three-Tesla magnetic resonance-guided prostate biopsy in men with increased prostate-specific antigen and repeated, negative, random, systematic, transrectal ultrasound biopsies: detection of clinically significant prostate cancers. Eur Urol 2012;62(5): 902–9.

30. Marks L, Young S, Natarajan S. MRI-ultrasound fusion for guidance of targeted prostate biopsy. Curr Opin Urol 2013;23(1):43–50.

31. Overduin CG, Futterer JJ, Barentsz JO. MRI-guided biopsy for prostate cancer detection: a systematic review of current clinical results. Curr Urol Rep 2013;14(3):209–13.

32. Reynier C, Troccaz J, Fourneret P, et al. MRI/TRUS data fusion for prostate brachytherapy. Preliminary results. Med Phys 2004;31(6):1568–75.

33. Schlaier JR, Warnat J, Dorenbeck U, et al. Image fusion of MR images and real-time ultrasonography: evaluation of fusion accuracy combining two commercial instruments, a neuronavigation system and a ultrasound system. Acta Neurochir 2004;146(3): 271–6 [discussion: 276–7].

34. Smeenge M, de la Rosette JJ, Wijkstra H. Current status of transrectal ultrasound techniques in prostate cancer. Curr Opin Urol 2012;22(4):297–302.

35. Hossack T, Patel MI, Huo A, et al. Location and pathological characteristics of cancers in radical prostatectomy specimens identified by transperineal biopsy compared to transrectal biopsy. J Urol 2012;188(3):781–5.

36. Lawrentschuk N, Haider MA, Daljeet N, et al. 'Prostatic evasive anterior tumours': the role of magnetic resonance imaging. BJU Int 2010;105(9):1231–6.

37. Mabjeesh NJ, Lidawi G, Chen J, et al. High detection rate of significant prostate tumours in anterior zones using transperineal ultrasound-guided template saturation biopsy. BJU Int 2012;110(7):993–7.

38. Rosset A, Spadola L, Ratib O. OsiriX: an open-source software for navigating in multidimensional DICOM images. J Digit Imaging 2004;17(3):205–16.

39. Adamy A, Yee DS, Matsushita K, et al. Role of prostate specific antigen and immediate confirmatory biopsy in predicting progression during active surveillance for low risk prostate cancer. J Urol 2011;185(2):477–82.

40. Barzell WE, Melamed MR, Cathcart P, et al. Identifying candidates for active surveillance: an evaluation of the repeat biopsy strategy for men with favorable risk prostate cancer. J Urol 2012;188(3):762–7.

41. Dall'Era MA, Albertsen PC, Bangma C, et al. Active surveillance for prostate cancer: a systematic review of the literature. Eur Urol 2012;62(6):976–83.

42. Ukimura O, Hirahara N, Fujihara A, et al. Technique for a hybrid system of real-time transrectal ultrasound with preoperative magnetic resonance imaging in the guidance of targeted prostate biopsy. Int J Urol 2010;17(10):890–3.

43. Xu S, Kruecker J, Guion P, et al. Closed-loop control in fused MR-TRUS image-guided prostate biopsy. Med Image Comput Comput Assist Interv 2007; 10(Pt 1):128–35.

44. Pinto PA, Chung PH, Rastinehad AR, et al. Magnetic resonance imaging/ultrasound fusion guided prostate biopsy improves cancer detection following transrectal ultrasound biopsy and correlates with multiparametric magnetic resonance imaging. J Urol 2011;186(4):1281–5.

45. Miyagawa T, Ishikawa S, Kimura T, et al. Real-time virtual sonography for navigation during targeted prostate biopsy using magnetic resonance imaging data. Int J Urol 2010;17(10):855–60.

46. Ukimura O, Desai MM, Palmer S, et al. 3-Dimensional elastic registration system of prostate biopsy location by real-time 3-dimensional transrectal ultrasound guidance with magnetic resonance/transrectal ultrasound image fusion. J Urol 2012;187(3): 1080–6.

47. Natarajan S, Marks LS, Margolis DJ, et al. Clinical application of a 3D ultrasound-guided prostate biopsy system. Urol Oncol 2011;29(3):334–42.

48. Bax J, Cool D, Gardi L, et al. Mechanically assisted 3D ultrasound guided prostate biopsy system. Med Phys 2008;35(12):5397–410.

49. Narayanan RK, Shinohara K, Crawford ED, et al. MRI-ultrasound registration for targeted prostate biopsy. Paper presented at: ISBI'09 Proceedings of the Sixth IEEE international conference on Symposium on Biomedical Imaging. From Nano to Macro. Boston, June 28–July 9, 2009.

Diffusion-Weighted Imaging of the Male Pelvis

Rahul A. Sheth, MD[a], Leonardo K. Bittencourt, MD, PhD[b],
Alexander R. Guimaraes, MD, PhD[c],*

KEYWORDS

• Diffusion-weighted imaging • Male pelvis • Magnetic resonance imaging • Cancer

KEY POINTS

- Diffusion-weighted (DW) imaging is playing an increasingly important role in disease detection, prognostication, and monitoring of treatment response. Particularly in the realm of oncology, the potential applications for DW imaging continue to expand.
- As magnetic resonance (MR) imaging plays a role in the diagnosis, characterization, and staging of most of these diseases, and DW imaging is a noninvasive, robust tool, its added value is only beginning to be realized.
- DW imaging holds promise for providing earlier cancer detection and evaluation of the treatment response. DW imaging enjoys several advantages over other advanced MR imaging tools, including the lack of reliance on intravenous contrast and relative rapidity of image acquisition.

INTRODUCTION

Diffusion-weighted (DW) imaging is playing an increasingly important role in disease detection, prognostication, and monitoring of treatment response. Particularly in the realm of oncology, the potential applications for DW imaging continue to expand. This technique has been applied toward the detection and characterization of a wide range of primary malignancies. It has also shown particular utility in the noninvasive staging of cancers. In addition, DW imaging holds promise for providing earlier cancer detection and evaluation of treatment response. DW imaging enjoys several advantages over other advanced magnetic resonance (MR) imaging tools, including lack of reliance on intravenous contrast and relative rapidity of image acquisition. As a quantitative imaging tool, DW imaging may also provide important information regarding tumor aggressiveness and histologic grading in a noninvasive manner.

In this article, the authors detail the role of DW imaging for pathologic processes involving the male pelvis. The authors describe the current data, new insights, and ongoing controversies regarding DW imaging of the male pelvis with a particular emphasis on oncologic applications. The authors also discuss imaging techniques and common pitfalls for DW imaging in this anatomic region.

TECHNIQUE
Principles of DW Imaging

Signal intensity in DW imaging is predicated on the relative freedom by which water molecules are able to move within tissue. In an unrestricted system, water molecules move randomly, a property initially observed in the 1800s and later mathematically characterized by Albert Einstein in 1905. Water within tissue, on the other hand, cannot move in an entirely random manner. Intracellular water is

Disclosures: none.
[a] Department of Radiology, Massachusetts General Hospital, 55 Fruit Street, Boston, MA 02114, USA;
[b] Abdominal and Pelvic Imaging, Clinica de Diagnostico por Imagem (CDPI), Department of Radiology, Rio de Janeiro Federal University, Av das Americas 4666, Sala 325, Rio de Janeiro 22640902, Brazil; [c] Martinos Center for Biomedical Imaging, Department of Radiology, Massachusetts General Hospital, Charlestown, MA 02129, USA
* Corresponding author.
E-mail address: aguimaraes@mgh.harvard.edu

Magn Reson Imaging Clin N Am 22 (2014) 145–163
http://dx.doi.org/10.1016/j.mric.2014.01.003
1064-9689/14/$ – see front matter © 2014 Elsevier Inc. All rights reserved

obstructed by organelles within the cell and the plasma membrane constraining the cellular contents; likewise, the motion of extracellular water is limited by extracellular matrix and cell membranes. Tissues with high cellularity, therefore, restrict the motion of water to a greater degree than tissues with low cellularity or tissues consisting of cells with defective plasma membranes.[1]

DW imaging as an MR imaging technique has its roots in 1965, when it was conceived as a variation of a T2-weighted pulse sequence.[2] The value of this imaging technique to identify areas of acute infarction in the brain led to its widespread use in neuroimaging. However, more recently, its relevance toward pelvic imaging has begun to be appreciated. This new appreciation is possible in part because of technological advances in the 1990s, including the development of stronger diffusion gradients and faster imaging sequences.[1,3]

Technical Aspects of DW Imaging

Imaging of the pelvis with MR imaging can be challenging because of the susceptibility artifact created at multiple air-tissue interfaces. Moreover, bowel motion can degrade image quality. Some institutions routinely administer spasmolytic drugs to inhibit peristalsis. Also, though not commonly performed, a homogenous material, such as ultrasound gel, can be used to fill the rectum to reduce the susceptibility signal caused by air in the rectum. DW imaging is typically performed in the axial plane, as the magnetic field homogeneity is best at the isocenter of the bore in addition to reducing eddy currents. However, for certain applications, such as rectal imaging, acquiring images in an oblique plane orthogonal to the long axis of the organ under investigation may facilitate evaluation of the extent of disease spread. Respiratory motion is not a common problem in pelvic imaging, though in some patients respiratory-triggered imaging may improve image resolution.[4]

DW imaging can be performed at either 1.5T or 3.0T, with the higher magnetic field strength offering higher signal to noise, though at the expense of worse susceptibility artifacts. In DW imaging, 2 symmetric gradients are applied on either side temporally of the 180° refocusing radiofrequency pulse of a conventional spin-echo T2-weighted sequence. The effects of the first gradient, known as the *dephasing gradient*, are nullified by the second gradient, known as the *rephasing gradient*, in tissues with protons whose free movement is restricted. The net effect on the transverse magnetization is, therefore, minimal, and there is no signal loss. On the other hand, protons that are freely moving within the tissue will experience

different strengths of the 2 gradients, and so the net effect will not be zero; these protons will not be fully rephased, resulting in signal loss. The 2 diffusion gradients are characterized by a constant b, which encapsulates the strength, duration, and time interval between the 2 gradients and is measured in units of seconds per square millimeter. At b = 0, a DW imaging pulse sequence is simply a T2-weighted imaging sequence. As the b value increases, the relative contribution of tissue diffusivity to signal intensity increases. Areas of restricted diffusion will appear bright on high b-value images, whereas areas of free-flowing fluid, such as within cysts or within the bladder, will appear dark.

Diffusivity of tissue can be quantified using DW imaging by calculating a value known as the *apparent diffusion coefficient* (ADC). The ADC is calculated as the slope of the line on a log linear plot connecting the signal intensity of a pixel measured at different b values; therefore, measurements of signal intensity from at least 2 b values are required, and the accuracy of the ADC value improves when more data points (ie, b values) are acquired. The choice of b value, however, to determine the ADC is a point of controversy, with low b values (10–150) being heavily weighted to perfusion effects (so-called intravoxel incoherent motion), and higher b values demonstrating improved diffusion weighting. As a result of the perfusion weighting, there is alteration of the expected mono-exponential behavior of signal loss with b-value increase, potentially altering calculated ADC values. There is growing consensus about avoiding low b values (<150) when using mono-exponential fitting as a result of this added perfusion weighting, in addition to clearly visible nonlinear behavior on log-linear plots. The low b-value imaging, however, has excellent value in lesion detection secondary to its high signal-to-noise ratio. Until these data are better understood, it is recommended to use at least 3 to 4 b values less than 1000 in order to calculate ADC. Regardless, the ADC value is independent of magnetic field strength.

Interpretation of DW Imaging

The diffusivity of water is inversely proportional to the organization and compactness of a tissue's microenvironment. Three discrete tissue characterization patterns can be described in DW imaging. Malignant lesions, because of their dense cellularity and disordered interstitium, demonstrate restricted diffusion. Fluid or necrotic tissue in which the integrity of plasma membranes has been compromised, allow for the free diffusion of water and, therefore, have the opposite signal characteristics of tumors; that is, they are dark on high b-value images and bright on ADC maps. Finally, rapidly flowing water within blood vessels will appear dark even on low b-value images.[5]

Malignant lesions, because of their hypercellularity, restrict the free diffusion of water. This restriction manifests on DW imaging as high signal within lesions on images acquired at high b values (>800 s/mm^2). Likewise, these lesions appear as low signal intensity on the ADC maps.

Consideration of the ADC value of a suspected malignant lesion is of paramount importance, as lesions with intrinsic T2 hyperintensity may still appear bright on high b-value imaging but should appear bright on the ADC map, indicating T2 "shine-through." Moreover, the clinical context of the examination must be taken into account when interpreting lesions that demonstrate restricted diffusion, as tumors are not the only pathologic conditions that exhibit this tissue characteristic. For example, abscesses may appear bright at high b values as well as dark on ADC maps, and the patients' presenting symptoms may be the only guide to differentiate between malignancy and infection.[4] The distribution of restricted diffusion within the lesion can also guide differentiating between these two causes. That is, tumors tend to demonstrate peripheral restricted diffusion with central necrosis, akin to a chocolate donut on an ADC map with a dark outer component and a bright inner component; inversely, abscesses tend to demonstrate central restricted diffusion, resembling a vanilla donut on ADC maps.

Limitations of DW Imaging

Although DW imaging holds the promise of being a quantitative imaging tool, precision in the quantification of ADC maps remains a challenge in DW imaging. There remains wide variability in published ADC values for similar pathologic conditions.[6] This variability is likely caused by a multitude of factors. First, there is no standardized protocol for performing DW imaging, and parameters such as b values can differ significantly across institutions, rendering comparison of ADC values from different published reports fraught with peril. When imaging at higher b values, signal to noise can decrease, which in turn can degrade the quality of the data used to calculate ADC values. Moreover, as DW imaging is a variation on T2-weighted imaging, the parameters that affect the T2 signal will affect the DW imaging signal intensity. For example, the lack of fat-suppression techniques, parallel imaging, matrix size, and echo train length

may all affect the T2 signal intensity and, therefore, the ADC value.

The importance of quantitative analysis of ADC maps remains an area of controversy. In addition to the issues surrounding relatively low b values exhibiting added perfusion effects to diffusivity and thereby altering mono-exponential behavior and, therefore, the ADC value, an ADC value that can be used as a cutoff between malignancy and benignity is also a concept of wide variability and controversy, so much so that centralized efforts (eg, Quantitative Imaging Biomarkers Alliance, https://www.rsna.org/QIBA) using internal standards (eg, muscle) to gauge restriction are necessary.

Not all malignancies demonstrate restricted diffusion. For example, mucinous adenocarcinomas of the colon may not be bright on high b-value imaging; likewise, calcified lesions will appear as signal voids.[7] Additionally, not all lesions that demonstrate restricted diffusion are malignant. For example, abscesses and cytotoxic edema also classically demonstrate restricted diffusion. Finally, DW imaging is burdened by poor spatial resolution, which limits the detectability of tumors less than approximately 1 cm in size.[5]

PROSTATE
Specific Technical Considerations

Endorectal coils provide higher-quality imaging of the prostate and are used whenever possible, primarily for improved T2-weighted imaging. Given the intrinsically high T2 signal of the peripheral zone of the prostate, described in further detail later, a multiple b-value approach is generally taken, whereby data are acquired at several b values, such as b = 0, 50, 400, and 800 s/mm^2. Recent provocative results have identified possible utility in ultrahigh b-value imaging within the prostate gland, exploiting kurtosis as a means to better detect and characterize malignancy.[8] These data are then used to calculate a mono-exponential ADC map.

Prostate Cancer Imaging

Background
Prostate cancer is the most common malignancy in men and second most common cause of cancer-related deaths in men. Clinical suspicion for prostate cancer is typically raised by palpation of a firm nodule on digital rectal examination or an elevated serum prostate-specific antigen (PSA) level; however, it is important to note that not all prostate cancers are associated with an elevation in PSA. A typical evaluation for prostate cancer

includes a systematic 12 core prostate biopsy, commonly performed with transrectal ultrasound guidance. If the biopsy is positive for malignancy, the patients' treatment plan is tailored to their symptoms and their life expectancy. For symptomatic patients with greater than 5 years of life expectancy, pelvic imaging with computed tomography (CT) or MR imaging is recommended if the patients' biopsy revealed either T3/T4 disease or T1/T2 disease with a greater than 10% chance of lymph node metastasis. For these patients, imaging plays a key role in the identification of lymph node metastases.

For patients with very-low-risk disease and a life expectancy of greater than 20 years, or for those patients with low-risk disease and a life expectancy of less than 10 years, active surveillance is an increasingly used approach. These patients undergo routine PSA checks as well as other diagnostic tests to vigilantly monitor the disease and detect early signs of progression. If there is a clinical concern for disease progression, usually indicated by an elevated PSA, repeat prostate biopsy is performed. However, this procedure is an imperfect evaluation of the prostate, both because nontargeted cores are obtained and because the anterior prostate is inaccessible to transrectal sampling. Therefore, patients in this low-risk category undergo MR imaging, particularly to evaluate the anterior prostate. Indeed, MR imaging is more accurate than transrectal biopsy or digital rectal examination in identifying prostate cancer[9] and possibly better correlated to the actual tumor aggressiveness parameters.[10]

A third scenario in which MR imaging plays a role in the management of patients with prostate cancer is in the setting of biochemical recurrence following radical prostatectomy. That is, for patients with increasing PSA levels following radical prostatectomy, MR imaging may assist in identifying residual or recurrent foci of malignancy in the resection bed.

Prostate cancer typically develops in the peripheral zone of the prostate; on MR imaging, focal malignant lesions appear as low-signal-intensity areas on T2-weighted imaging, a feature that defines it against a background of typically high T2 signal in the peripheral gland tissue. However, not all areas of low T2 signal in the peripheral gland are malignant, as mimickers, including hemorrhage, prostatitis, and posttreatment change, may share a similar appearance. The challenge of arriving at a specific diagnosis for malignancy on conventional MR imaging is all the more difficult for the minority of tumors that arise in the central gland; this region of the prostate usually demonstrates a heterogeneous T2 appearance because

of the benign prostatic hyperplasia, and so the identification of a focal lesion within the morass of T2 signal variability is not trivial (**Fig. 1**).[1]

DW imaging of prostate cancer

DW imaging has been evaluated extensively as a tissue characterization tool to assist in the identification of prostate malignancy. On DW imaging, prostate cancer classically appears bright at high b values and is dark on ADC maps; this latter finding may be of value when attempting to identify a discrete lesion within areas of heterogeneous T2 signal. Evaluation for prostate cancer that includes both T2-weighted imaging and DW imaging is superior to evaluations that rely on T2-weighted imaging alone (**Fig. 2**).[11]

Multiple published series have highlighted the ability of DW imaging to define focal malignant lesions within the peripheral zone.[11–24] Reported sensitivities and specificities vary broadly across studies, ranging from 40% to 95% for either. DW imaging, when used in conjunction with T2-weighted imaging, both significantly improves the sensitivity and specificity for identifying prostate cancer in the peripheral zone and reduces interobserver variability.[11,12,16,17,19,23,25] A recent study by Mazaheri and colleagues[12] found a sensitivity of 82% and specificity of 95% using an ADC cutoff value of 1.6×10^{-3} mm^2/s. However, because of the lack of standardization of imaging parameters, comparison of such absolute ADC cutoff values between studies is limited.

DW imaging of the central gland is less specific for malignancy owing to the overlap in imaging appearances of cancer and benign prostatic hyperplasia.[13,17,21,26–29] In a study by Oto and colleagues,[30] 38 tumors were compared with 38 foci of stromal hyperplasia and 38 areas of glandular hyperplasia in the central gland; although the mean ADC values of these 3 groups were statistically significantly different, there was a high degree of overlap between the individual values. More recently, Hoeks and colleagues[31] retrospectively reviewed 3T MR imaging examinations performed with endorectal coils on patients who subsequently underwent prostatectomy. They found that dynamic contrast imaging and DW imaging did not improve on detection accuracy over T2-weighted imaging for transition zone tumors.

Patients enrolled in an active surveillance protocol with an increasing PSA level but negative transrectal prostate biopsy may significantly benefit from DW imaging. Park and colleagues[20] reported on 43 patients with negative prostate biopsies and persistently elevated PSA levels who underwent DW imaging before rebiopsy. DW imaging was used to localize the most

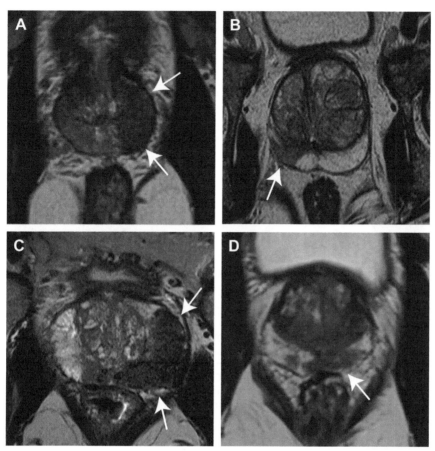

Fig. 1. Prostate cancer and its confounders on T2-weighted imaging. In a manner similar to prostate cancer (*A*), different lesions and conditions affecting the prostate may appear as focal T2-hypointense areas in the peripheral zone, as highlighted by the arrows in the images above. Examples include prostatitis (*B*), hemorrhage (*C*), and atrophy (*D*). This nonspecific appearance of prostate cancer lends credence to the importance of a multiparametric approach to prostate MR imaging, as accurate diagnosis requires integration of T2 signal characteristics as well as DW imaging, dynamic contrast-enhanced imaging, and/or spectroscopy.

suspicious area to be targeted by the subsequent biopsy; this location was defined as the area with the lowest ADC value. The researchers found that a significant portion of the cancers in their study group were in the transitional zone (76%), an area not routinely sampled in random prostate biopsies. Of the 17 cancers identified on DW imaging, only 6 were detectable on T2-weighted imaging alone. DW imaging, therefore, may be a powerful tool for biopsy guidance in patients with suspicion for malignancy but an initial negative biopsy.

DW imaging may play an increasingly important role in predicting prostate cancer aggressiveness. Although the histology-based Gleason grading system is a critical component in prognosticating disease-free survival, this method is inherently limited because it is based on a random sampling of prostate tissue. The biopsy-based Gleason score may significantly underestimate the final postprostatectomy score.[32] DW imaging could potentially fulfill the current unmet clinical need for accurate prediction of prostate cancer aggressiveness. Indeed, multiple studies have identified an inverse proportionality between ADC value and Gleason score, based on transrectal ultrasound-guided prostate biopsies, MR-guided prostate biopsies, or prostatectomy specimens.[10,33–38] However, there is a significant overlap of ADC values for different Gleason scores; so at present, an ADC value cannot be used to accurately estimate a Gleason score.

DW imaging has also been used to augment noninvasive prostate cancer staging, specifically with regard to involvement of the seminal vesicles. Invasion of the seminal vesicles by prostate cancer is an important negative prognostic indicator. Two reports[18,22] describe the ability of DW imaging to

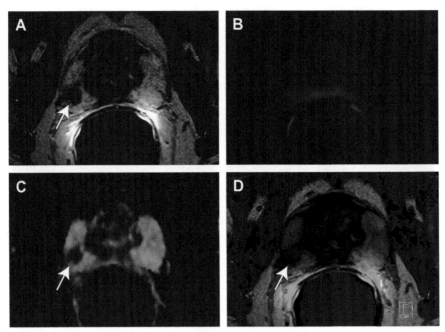

Fig. 2. Typical appearance of focal prostate cancer on DW imaging. Prostate cancer in the peripheral zone typically appears as a focal fusiform or oval-shaped lesion (*arrow*) with low signal intensity on T2-weighted imaging (*A*). Because DW images with b values less than 1000 s/mm² may not accurately discriminate between the lesion and background parenchyma (*B*), the calculation of ADC maps is mandatory (lesion highlighted by *arrow*) (*C*). In this case, the ADC map reveals restricted diffusion in the same location as the abnormality on T2-weighted imaging. Fusion imaging (*D*) overlaying the ADC data on the T2-weighted image provides both diffusion and anatomic information (lesion highlighted by *arrow*).

predict seminal vesicle involvement. When combined with T2-weighted imaging, DW imaging improved accuracy and specificity to approximately 97% and 96%, respectively, compared with T2-weighted imaging alone.

DW imaging has also been applied to the evaluation of treatment response in prostate cancer. For postradiation and post–high-intensity focused ultrasound therapy for prostate cancer, DW imaging improves on the detection of residual tumor compared with T2-weighted imaging alone (**Fig. 3**).[39,40] However, at present, there is insufficient evidence to rely on DW imaging alone for these patients; dynamic contrast-enhanced (DCE) MR imaging remains the imaging tool of choice in this setting.

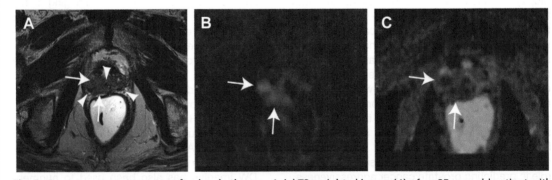

Fig. 3. Prostate cancer recurrence after brachytherapy. Axial T2-weighted image (*A*) of an 85-year-old patient with rising PSA levels after brachytherapy show the brachytherapy seeds as small T2 hypointense dots distributed throughout the gland (*arrowheads*). Although the parenchyma is diffusely heterogeneous, there is a somewhat discrete area with low signal intensity between 2 radioactive seeds resulting in a focal bulge along the capsular contour (*arrows*). DW imaging shows restricted diffusion in this area (*arrows*), with high signal intensity on b = 1000 s/mm² imaging (*B*) and low signal intensity (*arrows*) on the ADC map (*C*).

DW imaging has also shown utility in predicting patients who will exhibit biochemical recurrence following radical prostatectomy. In a retrospective study of 30 patients after surgical resection with elevated PSA, the presurgical ADC value of the tumor was the only independent predictive factor for biochemical recurrence.[41] Identifying the site of local recurrence can be challenging, but DW imaging also shows promise in this regard. Giannarini and colleagues[42] reported on a small case series of 5 patients for whom DW imaging was the only imaging modality able to identify the site of recurrence, all of which were confirmed histologically.

BLADDER
Specific Technical Considerations

Bladder distention is a prerequisite for MR imaging of the bladder. For patients with indwelling catheters, 250 to 400 mL of saline can be infused into the bladder. Otherwise, patients should be instructed to drink plenty of fluids before the examination. Care should be taken, however, to prevent overdistention of the bladder, as this can contribute to overstaging of bladder malignancy by MR imaging. As bladder filling is a dynamic process that can alter the morphology of the bladder during the MR imaging examination, it is important to be aware that lesions may seem to change location or shape during the course of the imaging study.

Bladder Cancer Imaging

Background
Bladder cancer is the fourth most common cancer in the United States and is 3 times more common in men than in women. Accurately characterizing tumors as muscle invasive versus superficial is of paramount clinical significance in bladder cancer. Tumors that only involve the subepithelial connective tissue are considered T1 lesions and are treated with transurethral resection of bladder tumor with or without adjuvant chemotherapy, followed by surveillance. On the other hand, T2 lesions that invade the muscularis propria are usually managed with a radical cystectomy. Accurate characterization of tumor invasiveness can have a profound impact on a patient's management.

MR imaging is commonly used for bladder cancer staging. However, this approach is not without its drawbacks. Specifically, MR imaging may overstage bladder cancer.[43] Moreover, contrast-enhanced imaging is an important component of the conventional MR evaluation of bladder cancer invasiveness; patients with impaired renal function may not be able to receive gadolinium-based contrast agents. DW imaging has, therefore, emerged as a potential alternative approach to contrast-enhanced MR imaging for bladder cancer detection, staging, and treatment monitoring. Because the median age at diagnosis of bladder cancer is 65 years, it is not uncommon for patients with this disease to have multiple medical comorbidities, including renal dysfunction that may preclude the use of gadolinium-based contrast agents.

DW imaging of bladder cancer
On high b-value imaging, bladder malignancies appear as bright lesions, well delineated along their luminal margin by the dark urine within the bladder.[44] The bladder wall has intrinsically intermediate signal intensity on high b-value images. On ADC maps, the tumors are dark, whereas normal bladder wall maintains an intermediate signal intensity (**Fig. 4**). Takeuchi and colleagues[45] studied the potential benefits of adding DW imaging to conventional T2-weighted imaging on accurately assessing bladder cancer staging. A total of 40 patients with 52 bladder malignancies underwent pelvic MR imaging before cystoscopy and tumor resection/sampling. The researchers compared the accuracy of tumor staging based on T2-weighted imaging alone, T2-weighted imaging with DW imaging, T2-weighted imaging with post–contrast-enhanced imaging, and all 3 combined; they found the respective accuracies to be 67%, 88%, 79%, and 92%. The tissue characterization of DW imaging augmented the accuracy of the T2-weighted imaging interpretation to a greater degree than postcontrast imaging. There was a statistically significant improvement in specificity and area under the receiver operating characteristic (ROC) curve by adding DW imaging to T2-weighted imaging. The researchers also conceived a useful system of morphologic descriptors for bladder cancer that predicts tumor staging. Tumors that are T1 may be flat or demonstrate an inchworm appearance, with a C-shaped tumor enveloping a submucosal stalk. Tumors that extend into the submucosa but with smooth margins are likely to be T2, whereas tumors with irregular spiculations extending into the bladder wall are likely T3 or greater.

Likewise, Abou-El-Ghar and colleagues[44] showed that DW imaging was able to accurately differentiate 106 malignant bladder lesions from 14 nonmalignant causes of hematuria, though the added benefit of DW imaging over T2-weighted imaging was small; the marginal benefit was likely biased by the large size of the malignant lesions.

DW imaging may also be capable of predicting the aggressiveness of bladder cancers. Kobayashi and colleagues[46] calculated ADC values for 104 bladder tumors and compared the imaging

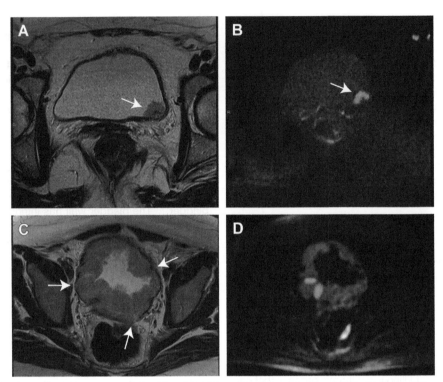

Fig. 4. Muscle-sparing versus muscle-invasive transitional cell carcinoma of the bladder. (*A*) and (*B*) are T2-weighted and DW images, respectively, of a 52-year-old female patient and are notable for a T2 hyperintense polypoid lesion (*arrow*) along the posterolateral left bladder wall with associated restricted diffusion and with a classic inchworm morphology. Conversely, (*C*) and (*D*) are T2 and DW images, respectively, of a 74-year-old patient and are significant for diffuse irregular thickening of the bladder wall (*arrows*), with several focal areas of interruption of the usually T2 hypointense muscular layer, raising the suspicion for muscular invasion. DW imaging shows restricted diffusion throughout the circumferential lesion.

findings with the histologic T stage and grade. Tumors classified as T1 or T2 demonstrated statistically significantly lower ADC values than low-grade tumors, such as noninvasive papillary carcinomas. Moreover, histologically high-grade tumors were also found to have statistically significantly higher ADC values than low-grade tumors. These data suggest that quantitative DW imaging could provide foresight into bladder cancer aggressiveness.

DW imaging may also serve as a predictor for the response to chemotherapy in bladder cancer. Although radical cystectomy is the standard of care for patients with muscle-invasive bladder cancer, bladder-sparing protocols are being actively explored to preserve patients' quality of life. The selection of patients who would be eligible for bladder preservation rests heavily on determining whether patients achieved a complete response to induction chemoradiation therapy, and so the accurate determination of residual tumor in these patients is crucial. Differentiating residual tumor from posttreatment fibrosis,

particularly following transurethral resection and radiation therapy, however, is not necessarily straightforward on conventional MR imaging (**Fig. 5**). Postsurgical and postradiation changes both appear as areas of bladder wall thickening with intramural T2 hyperintense signal. Postcontrast imaging, although an improvement, may also be misleading: contrast can accumulate in areas of residual cancer or inflammation. Yoshida and colleagues[47] investigated the ability of DW imaging to predict residual tumor following chemoradiation and before surgical excision. They prospectively enrolled 20 patients with muscle-invasive bladder cancer who had undergone debulking transurethral resection. Imaging was performed 4 to 6 weeks following the completion of a course of chemoradiation therapy. Following the MR examination, the patients underwent either partial or radical cystectomy; the histologic result for residual tumor or complete response was used as the gold standard. The researchers found a dramatic increase in specificity and accuracy for predicting complete response with DW imaging

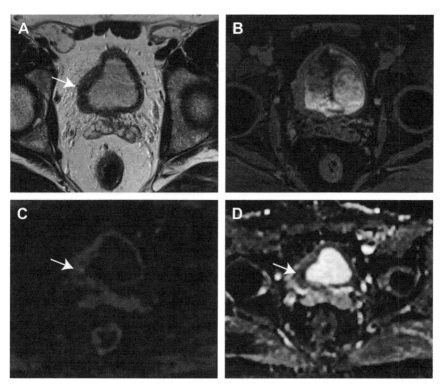

Fig. 5. Flat transitional cell carcinoma of the bladder wall visualized on DW imaging. T2-weighted imaging (*A*) shows mild thickening of the right bladder wall (*arrow*), with homogenous low signal intensity consistent with scarring from prior transurethral resection of a bladder wall tumor. Postcontrast T1-weighted images (*B*) show no evidence of abnormal enhancement in the thickened wall. However, on DW imaging with b = 1000 s/mm^2 (*C*), there is a focal area of high signal intensity (*arrow*), which shows restricted diffusion on the ADC map (*D*). A focal high-grade invasive transitional cell carcinoma of the bladder was identified on subsequent cystoscopy and biopsy in this location (*arrow*).

(92% and 80%, respectively) compared with T2-weighted imaging and contrast-enhanced MR imaging. If validation of bladder-sparing protocols occurs following randomized trials, DW imaging could represent an integral component of patient selection.

BOWEL AND RECTUM
Rectal Cancer

Introduction
Colorectal cancer is the fourth most common cancer in the United States and the second most common cause of cancer-related death. As with bladder cancer, the clinical stage of rectal cancer drives the decision-making process for determining a patient's treatment course; imaging plays a central role in this process. MR imaging of the pelvis is a recommended examination for all patients with potentially surgically resectable rectal cancers to provide a preoperative assessment of the depth of tumor infiltration into the rectal wall and to identify pelvic lymph node metastases.

DW imaging of rectal cancer
Conventional MR imaging is very effective at predicting the presence of muscularis propria invasion, with a reported sensitivity of approximately 94%.[48] In some instances, though, DW imaging can assist in making the diagnosis of rectal cancer. For example, T2-weighted imaging of rectal cancer can be challenging because both normal mucosa and malignant tissue may be similarly hyperintense. On high b-value DW imaging, however, the signal intensity of normal mucosa decreases, whereas malignant lesions remain hyperintense (**Fig. 6**). Indeed, in a study of 45 patients with rectal cancer, Rao and colleagues[49] showed that the addition of DW imaging to T2-weighted imaging increased the area under the ROC curve from 0.93 to 0.99.

Although there is little room for improvement in determining a cancer's T staging with conventional MR imaging, DW imaging has been successfully applied to increasing the performance of MR in predicting the response to chemoradiation therapy and in characterizing the circumferential

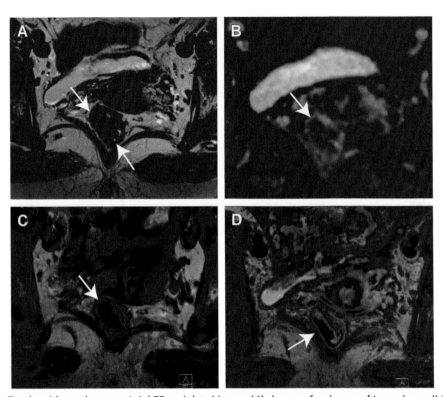

Fig. 6. Small polypoid rectal cancer. Axial T2-weighted image (*A*) shows a focal area of irregular wall thickening involving the posterolateral right aspect of the middle third of the rectum (*arrows*). ADC map (*B*) shows restricted diffusion (*arrow*), and fusion of the DW imaging with the T2 image (*C*) demonstrates colocalization of the abnormality (*arrow*). DCE imaging (*D*) also shows a focal hot spot of early enhancement within this lesion (*arrow*).

resection margin. Neoadjuvant chemoradiation therapy is administered to patients with stage II and III rectal cancer because of the risk of locoregional recurrence following surgery. A significant proportion of patients are subsequently downstaged following preoperative therapy, and approximately 20% of patients show complete response.[50–56] In the MERCURY trial, a prospective study of 111 patients, tumor regression as assessed by MR imaging, is a strong predictor of overall and disease-free survival.[57] Therefore, the ability to noninvasively track the response to therapy with MR imaging could potentially provide powerful prognostic information. Moreover, complete response on imaging could potentially obviate surgery at all, though this approach has yet to be rigorously tested in a clinical trial.

One drawback to conventional MR imaging's characterization of residual malignancy is the similar signal characteristics of tumor and post-treatment fibrosis.[58–60] On DW imaging, however, only tumor would be expected to demonstrate restricted diffusivity of water and could theoretically be differentiated from scar tissue. Kim and colleagues[61] reported in a study of 40 patients

who underwent neoadjuvant chemoradiation a significant improvement in the diagnostic accuracy of MR imaging when DW images were used to augment conventional T2-weighted images. The researchers found a statistically significantly lower ADC value in patients with residual tumor compared with those found to have a complete response at surgery (**Fig. 7**).

Moreover, DW imaging may be able to predict the response to therapy not only after the completion of chemoradiation but also possibly before or early within the treatment course. In a prospective study of 37 patients, Sun and colleagues[62] performed DW imaging before the initiation of neoadjuvant chemoradiation therapy, after the first week of therapy, after the second week of therapy, and before surgery. The ADC values for the tumors were calculated at each time point, and the efficacy of preoperative therapy was determined by histologic analysis of the surgical specimen. The researchers found a statistically significantly lower mean tumor ADC value in tumors that were downstaged at surgery compared with those that were not on the pretreatment MR examination. The downstaged tumors also demonstrated

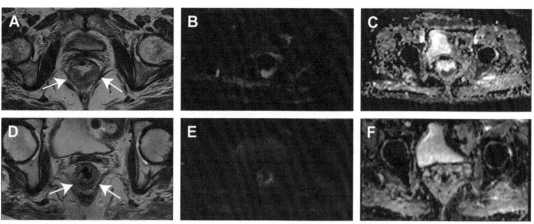

Fig. 7. Pretreatment (A–C) and posttreatment (D–F) MR images of an 84-year-old female patient with rectal cancer treated with chemoradiation. Axial T2-weighted images (A, D) show a marked reduction in size of the focal irregular thickening involving the posterior rectal wall (arrows). This area appears as a linear, low-signal intensity lesion on the posttreatment image (D). Pretreatment DW imaging shows marked restricted diffusion (B, C) within the lesion. Although this area is mildly persistently hyperintense on posttreatment DW imaging (E), the interval increase in ADC value (F) indicates treatment response and fibrosis rather than residual tumor.

a significant increase in ADC value after 1 week of therapy, whereas the tumors that were not downstaged had ADC values that were unchanged compared with the pretreatment MR imaging. Likewise, Lambregts and colleagues[63] found, in a multicenter study of 120 patients, that the addition of DW imaging to conventional MR imaging improved radiologist accuracy at determining the complete response. DW imaging may also provide a better assessment of residual tumor viability than positron emission tomography (PET)-CT.[64] These data suggest that DW imaging could represent a biomarker for predicting the response to therapy, both a priori and early within the presurgical treatment course.

Beyond improving detection and predicting the response to chemoradiation, DW imaging has also been applied to rectal cancer for the assessment of the mesorectal fascia. A critical pathologic staging parameter in rectal cancer is the circumferential resection margin, a distance defined as the closest radial margin between the deepest component of the tumor and mesorectal fascia. A circumferential resection margin that is less than or equal to 1 mm is considered positive and portends a negative prognosis. In a meta-analysis of imaging modalities, conventional MR was estimated to have rather low sensitivity (82%) and specificity (76%) for identifying invasion of the mesorectal fascia; this is related to the apparent similarity between postradiation fibrosis and residual tumor on T2-weighted imaging. Park and colleagues[65] performed a retrospective study of 45 patients who received neoadjuvant

chemoradiation followed by surgery for rectal cancer. The ability of 2 independent readers to identify invasion of the mesorectal fascia by T2-weighted imaging alone or in combination with DW imaging was determined, with the surgical specimen serving as the gold standard. The additional information provided by DW imaging improved the diagnostic performance of both readers: accuracy of interpretation with both T2-weighted imaging and DW imaging was 89% and 93%.

Recent studies, however, have demonstrated improved preoperative staging by using fluorodeoxyglucose (FDG)-PET/CT in rectal cancer staging. In a prospective study, automatically generated PET/CT-based contours showed the best correlation with the surgical specimen and, thus, provided a useful and powerful tool to accurately determine the largest tumor dimension in rectal cancer. As these studies used fused MR and PET/CT data analysis, it is important to better understand the role that each of these modalities might play in primary staging of rectal cancer. Furthermore, FDG-PET/CT has played a role in diagnosing lymph node involvement; but as microscopic involvement of a lymph node becomes more accessible, the size sensitivity of FDG-PET becomes a problem. DW imaging–MR imaging has also played a role in determining nodal involvement in rectal cancer staging with limited sensitivity and specificity.[48,66–69]

PET/MR imaging could answer questions that have not been adequately answered, such as which modality individually is better for nodal staging. Moreover, the combination of two imaging modalities, by merging the whole-body imaging capabilities of PET with the spatial resolution of MRI, could provide the most definitive, accurate, and sensitive examination, all in one sitting (**Fig. 8**).

Inflammatory Bowel Disease

Background

Radiologic techniques play an integral role in the diagnosis and management of patients with inflammatory bowel disease (IBD). Imaging now not only assists in making the diagnosis of IBD, including helping to discriminate between ulcerative colitis (UC) and Crohn disease, but is also a critical component in the determination of active versus indolent disease. Imaging assessment of IBD activity is increasingly being used by surgeons and gastroenterologists for treatment planning and as a biomarker of treatment response/resistance.

DW imaging of IBD

A principal clinical question for which imaging is used in IBD is the determination of active versus inactive disease in the small bowel. This distinction is of high clinical significance: patients with active inflammation are treated medically with immunomodulatory therapy, whereas symptomatic patients with inactive, fibrosed strictures often require surgical intervention. Areas of actively inflamed bowel most commonly demonstrate pathologic bowel thickening, which is defined as a bowel wall greater than 3 mm in thickness. A 3-mm cutoff was selected by consensus as the best compromise between sensitivity and specificity and is, for the most part, used universally for all cross-sectional modalities. Another differentiating characteristic of active disease is mucosal hyperenhancement, which appears as a pencil-thin line outlining the luminal surface of the bowel wall and reflects the hyperemia of inflammation.

Although conventional MR enjoys a relatively high sensitivity for detecting active small bowel IBD,[70] the classic findings that differentiate active versus chronic inflammation may not always be present. Both active Crohn disease and UC manifest as lymphocytic infiltration and aggregation within the lamina propria and submucosa of the

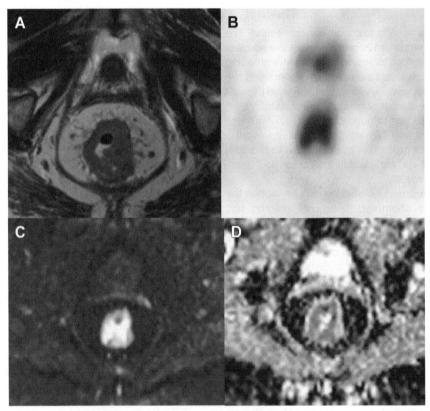

Fig. 8. MR positron emission tomography (PET) imaging of a T3 rectal cancer. Axial T2-weighted imaging (*A*) demonstrates a bulky mass with transmural extension into the mesorectal fascia. This mass demonstrates fluorodeoxyglucose avidity (*B*) and is hyperintense on DW imaging (*C*) demonstrating restricted diffusion (*D*) on ADC. This information was obtained with a single examination on the new MR-PET hybrid imaging platform.

bowel. This increased cellularity, in turn, results in impaired diffusivity of water in tissues, a phenomenon that can subsequently be detected and measured using DW imaging (**Fig. 9**).[7,71] Oto and colleagues[72,73] reviewed MR enterography examinations that included DCE–MR imaging and DW imaging for 18 patients with Crohn disease who had pathologically confirmed active inflammatory disease involving the terminal ileum within 2 months of the imaging examination. The researchers found that both DCE–MR imaging and DW imaging were capable of differentiating between actively inflamed and normal small bowel. Areas of inflammation were found to have significantly lower ADC values compared with normal loops of bowel. DW imaging demonstrated a higher sensitivity than DCE–MR imaging for inflamed bowel and does not require the use of intravenous contrast.

DW imaging may also provide a noninvasive means of assessing large bowel inflammation. Although this segment of the alimentary tract is best visualized directly through colonoscopy, the bowel preparation required for this procedure can be particularly onerous to a patient population who at baseline live with abdominal discomfort. Oussalah and colleagues[74] performed DW imaging of the colon in 96 patients, most of whom underwent colonoscopy within 48 hours of the imaging study. The study group included patients with Crohn disease and UC who clinically presented with acute inflammatory flares. No bowel preparation was administered to patients before the MR imaging, whereas standard bowel preparation was performed before colonoscopy. The researchers found that hyperintensity within colonic segments on high b-value images accurately predicted findings of inflammation on colonoscopy for both UC and Crohn disease. Thus, although it is unlikely that DW imaging will supplant colonoscopy, it may be a useful correlative tool in patients who are unable to tolerate the bowel preparation and/or the endoscopic procedure.

PENIS
Technique

Intracavernosal agents to cause tumescence are an important consideration for penile imaging. Tumescence allows for more uniform signal characteristics of the corpora, and it also facilitates positioning in the midline of patients.

Penile Cancer

There is no significant literature regarding the use of DW imaging for the detection or staging of penile cancer. However, most penile cancers are squamous cell carcinomas that share similar microenvironmental characteristics of other carcinomas, including hypercellularity and increased nuclear-to-cytoplasmic ratios. These characteristics, in turn, result in restricted diffusion of intracellular and interstitial water, which can be imaged with DW imaging (**Fig. 10**).[75] Likewise, infectious processes, such as abscesses, will appear dark on ADC maps (**Fig. 11**).

TESTES

As with the penis, there are limited amounts of data regarding the use of DW imaging of the testes. Ultrasonography remains the mainstay imaging modality for the scrotum and its contents. However, DW imaging may add value to conventional MR imaging for differentiating between benign and malignant testicular masses. This differentiation may be of vital importance for patients, as a confident diagnosis of a benign mass can spare patients from undergoing a radical orchiectomy. Tsili and colleagues,[76] in a small

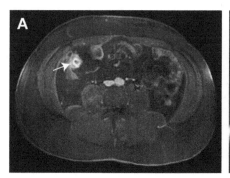
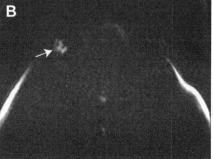

Fig. 9. DW imaging of active Crohn disease. Postcontrast T1-weighted (*A*) and DW (*B*) imaging from an MR enterography study of a child with Crohn disease. There is mural thickening and mucosal hyperenhancement involving the terminal ileum with associated restricted diffusion (*arrows*), consistent with active inflammation.

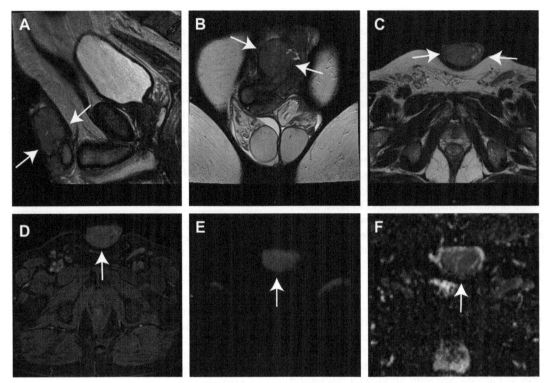

Fig. 10. MR imaging of penile cancer. Sagittal (*A*), coronal (*B*), and axial (*C*) T2-weighted imaging reveal an expansile, infiltrative mass with irregular margins (*arrows*), invading into the corpora cavernosa and spongiosum. The lesion (*arrows*) shows heterogeneous enhancement on postcontrast T1-weighted imaging (*D*) as well as high signal intensity on b = 1000 s/mm^2 DW imaging (*E*) and low ADC values (*F*).

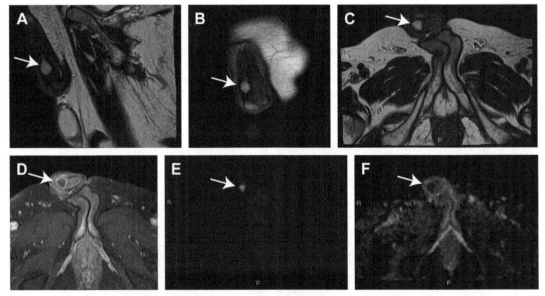

Fig. 11. Penile abscess caused by intracavernous papaverine injections. Sagittal (*A*), coronal (*B*), and axial (*C*) T2-weighted images show a well-defined ovoid fluid collection in the right corpus cavernosum (*arrows*). The collection (*arrow*) demonstrates peripheral contrast enhancement on T1-weighted imaging (*D*). DW imaging confirms that the collection (*arrow*) is an abscess by demonstrating internal restricted diffusion (*E*, *F*).

retrospective study of 26 men, found that benign testicular masses could be differentiated from normal testicular parenchyma based on their ADC value; moreover, malignant intratesticular masses were found to have a statistically significantly lower ADC value than benign intratesticular masses.

Additionally, DW imaging has been applied to the imaging of nononcologic processes. For example, Kantarci and colleagues[77] evaluated the added benefit of performed DW imaging during MR imaging evaluations for nonpalpable undescended testes. In a cohort of 36 boys who subsequently underwent laparoscopy after MR imaging, 2 readers were able to improve their accuracy of detecting the undescended testes with the addition of DW imaging from 86% and 84% to 92% and 86%, respectively.

LYMPH NODES

The presence of lymph node metastases greatly alters the treatment options as well as prognosis for patients with pelvic malignancies. Currently, there is no ideal test for differentiating between benign and malignant lymph nodes. To date, the most promising imaging technique to make this distinction, especially in the pelvis, is MR imaging enhanced with macrophage-specific iron oxide nanoparticles.[78] Lymph node size, particularly in the pelvis, is a poor indicator of malignant involvement. DW imaging has been applied toward the characterization of pelvic lymph nodes (**Fig. 12**).

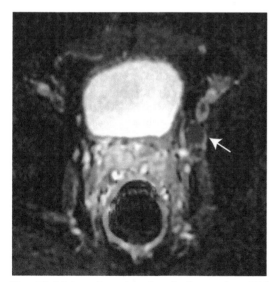

Fig. 12. Metastatic pelvic lymphadenopathy. ADC map in a patient with prostate cancer reveals a low ADC value for an enlarged left pelvic sidewall lymph node (*arrow*), consistent with metastasis.

In a study of 129 consecutive patients with rectal cancer who underwent preoperative MR imaging, Mizukami and colleagues[79] found a 93% negative predictive value of DW imaging for lymph node metastasis. The researchers characterized lymph nodes identified on T1- or T2-weighted images that were hyperintense on high b-value DW images as positive for metastatic deposits and those that were hypointense as negative. They found that DW imaging was highly accurate in predicting benign lymph nodes. The ability of DW imaging to accurately stage patients with rectal cancer as N0 has direct ramifications on clinical care, as patients with node-negative disease and no evidence of muscularis propria invasion by the primary tumor may be candidates for a less invasive, transanal curative surgery. However, the researchers in this study also noted a relatively high false-positive rate (14%); that is, a significant number of positive lymph nodes were found to be, in fact, reactive rather than malignant, a limitation of DW imaging that can lead to overstaging. Also, the characterization of lymph nodes by DW imaging is controversial, with recent data suggesting that ADC values cannot meaningfully differentiate between benign and malignant lymph nodes.[80]

In summary, DW imaging has a significant amount of added value to imaging oncologic and inflammatory processes affecting the male pelvis. As MR imaging plays a role in the diagnosis, characterization, and staging of most of these diseases, and DW imaging is a noninvasive, robust tool, its added value is only beginning to be realized. It is certain at this time that DW imaging is a valuable source of contrast and function aiding to the certainty of diagnoses in these conditions. As novel techniques, such as PET/MR imaging, come to fruition, a better understanding of the biophysical nature of this contrast mechanism and its relationship to other oncologic/inflammatory biomarkers (eg, FDG avidity) will be straightforward to study.

REFERENCES

1. Qayyum A. Diffusion-weighted imaging in the abdomen and pelvis: concepts and applications. Radiographics 2009;29(6):1797–810. http://dx.doi.org/10.1148/rg.296095521.
2. Sørland G, Aksnes D, Gjerdåker L. A pulsed field gradient spin-echo method for diffusion measurements in the presence of internal gradients. J Magn Reson 1999;137(2):397–401. http://dx.doi.org/10.1006/jmre.1998.1670.
3. Bittencourt LK, Matos C, Coutinho AC. Diffusion-weighted magnetic resonance imaging in the

upper abdomen: technical issues and clinical applications. Magn Reson Imaging Clin N Am 2011; 19(1):111–31. http://dx.doi.org/10.1016/j.mric.2010.09.002.

4. Thoeny HC, Forstner R, De Keyzer F. Genitourinary applications of diffusion-weighted MR imaging in the pelvis. Radiology 2012;263(2):326–42. http://dx.doi.org/10.1148/radiol.12110446.

5. Lim KS, Tan CH. Diffusion-weighted MRI of adult male pelvic cancers. Clin Radiol 2012; 67(9):899–908. http://dx.doi.org/10.1016/j.crad.2012.01.016.

6. Zhang JL, Sigmund EE, Chandarana H, et al. Variability of renal apparent diffusion coefficients: limitations of the monoexponential model for diffusion quantification. Radiology 2010;254(3):783–92. http://dx.doi.org/10.1148/radiol.09090891.

7. Sinha R, Rajiah P, Ramachandran I, et al. Diffusion-weighted MR imaging of the gastrointestinal tract: technique, indications, and imaging findings. Radiographics 2013;33(3):655–76. http://dx.doi.org/10.1148/rg.333125042 [discussion: 676–80].

8. Rosenkrantz AB, Sigmund EE, Johnson G, et al. Prostate cancer: feasibility and preliminary experience of a diffusional kurtosis model for detection and assessment of aggressiveness of peripheral zone cancer. Radiology 2012;264(1):126–35. http://dx.doi.org/10.1148/radiol.12112290.

9. Mullerad M, Hricak H, Kuroiwa K, et al. Comparison of endorectal magnetic resonance imaging, guided prostate biopsy and digital rectal examination in the preoperative anatomical localization of prostate cancer. J Urol 2005;174(6):2158–63. http://dx.doi.org/10.1097/01.ju.0000181224.95276.82.

10. Bittencourt LK, Barentsz JO, de Miranda LC, et al. Prostate MRI: diffusion-weighted imaging at 1.5T correlates better with prostatectomy Gleason grades than TRUS-guided biopsies in peripheral zone tumours. Eur Radiol 2012;22(2):468–75. http://dx.doi.org/10.1007/s00330-011-2269-1.

11. Haider MA, van der Kwast TH, Tanguay J, et al. Combined T2-weighted and diffusion-weighted MRI for localization of prostate cancer. AJR Am J Roentgenol 2007;189(2):323–8. http://dx.doi.org/10.2214/AJR.07.2211.

12. Mazaheri Y, Hricak H, Fine SW, et al. Prostate tumor volume measurement with combined T2-weighted imaging and diffusion-weighted MR: correlation with pathologic tumor volume. Radiology 2009; 252(2):449–57. http://dx.doi.org/10.1148/radiol.2523081423.

13. Tan CH, Wang J, Kundra V. Diffusion weighted imaging in prostate cancer. Eur Radiol 2011;21(3):593–603. http://dx.doi.org/10.1007/s00330-010-1960-y.

14. Tan CH, Wei W, Johnson V, et al. Diffusion-weighted MRI in the detection of prostate cancer: meta-analysis. AJR Am J Roentgenol 2012;199(4):822–9. http://dx.doi.org/10.2214/AJR.11.7805.

15. Morgan VA, Kyriazi S, Ashley SE, et al. Evaluation of the potential of diffusion-weighted imaging in prostate cancer detection. Acta Radiol 2007;48(6):695–703. http://dx.doi.org/10.1080/02841850701349257.

16. Miao H, Fukatsu H, Ishigaki T. Prostate cancer detection with 3-T MRI: comparison of diffusion-weighted and T2-weighted imaging. Eur J Radiol 2007;61(2):297–302. http://dx.doi.org/10.1016/j.ejrad.2006.10.002.

17. Yoshimitsu K, Kiyoshima K, Irie H, et al. Usefulness of apparent diffusion coefficient map in diagnosing prostate carcinoma: correlation with stepwise histopathology. J Magn Reson Imaging 2008;27(1):132–9. http://dx.doi.org/10.1002/jmri.21181.

18. Kim JH, Kim JK, Park BW, et al. Apparent diffusion coefficient: prostate cancer versus noncancerous tissue according to anatomical region. J Magn Reson Imaging 2008;28(5):1173–9. http://dx.doi.org/10.1002/jmri.21513.

19. Kajihara H, Hayashida Y, Murakami R, et al. Usefulness of diffusion-weighted imaging in the localization of prostate cancer. Int J Radiat Oncol Biol Phys 2009;74(2):399–403. http://dx.doi.org/10.1016/j.ijrobp.2008.08.017.

20. Park BK, Lee HM, Kim CK, et al. Lesion localization in patients with a previous negative transrectal ultrasound biopsy and persistently elevated prostate specific antigen level using diffusion-weighted imaging at three Tesla before rebiopsy. Invest Radiol 2008;43(11):789–93. http://dx.doi.org/10.1097/RLI.0b013e318183725e.

21. Shimofusa R, Fujimoto H, Akamata H, et al. Diffusion-weighted imaging of prostate cancer. J Comput Assist Tomogr 2005;29(2):149–53.

22. Ren J, Huan Y, Wang H, et al. Seminal vesicle invasion in prostate cancer: prediction with combined T2-weighted and diffusion-weighted MR imaging. Eur Radiol 2009;19(10):2481–6. http://dx.doi.org/10.1007/s00330-009-1428-0.

23. Lim HK, Kim JK, Kim KA, et al. Prostate cancer: apparent diffusion coefficient map with T2-weighted images for detection–a multireader study. Radiology 2009;250(1):145–51. http://dx.doi.org/10.1148/radiol.2501080207.

24. Kim CK, Choi D, Park BK, et al. Diffusion-weighted MR imaging for the evaluation of seminal vesicle invasion in prostate cancer: initial results. J Magn Reson Imaging 2008;28(4):963–9. http://dx.doi.org/10.1002/jmri.21531.

25. Tanimoto A, Nakashima J, Kohno H, et al. Prostate cancer screening: the clinical value of diffusion-weighted imaging and dynamic MR imaging in combination with T2-weighted imaging. J Magn Reson Imaging 2007;25(1):146–52. http://dx.doi.org/10.1002/jmri.20793.

26. Tamada T, Sone T, Toshimitsu S, et al. Age-related and zonal anatomical changes of apparent diffusion coefficient values in normal human prostatic tissues. J Magn Reson Imaging 2008;27(3):552–6. http://dx.doi.org/10.1002/jmri.21117.

27. Sato C, Naganawa S, Nakamura T, et al. Differentiation of noncancerous tissue and cancer lesions by apparent diffusion coefficient values in transition and peripheral zones of the prostate. J Magn Reson Imaging 2005;21(3):258–62. http://dx.doi.org/10.1002/jmri.20251.

28. Van As N, Charles-Edwards E, Jackson A, et al. Correlation of diffusion-weighted MRI with whole mount radical prostatectomy specimens. Br J Radiol 2008;81(966):456–62. http://dx.doi.org/10.1259/bjr/29869950.

29. Ren J, Huan Y, Wang H, et al. Diffusion-weighted imaging in normal prostate and differential diagnosis of prostate diseases. Abdom Imaging 2008;33(6):724–8. http://dx.doi.org/10.1007/s00261-008-9361-2.

30. Oto A, Kayhan A, Jiang Y, et al. Prostate cancer: differentiation of central gland cancer from benign prostatic hyperplasia by using diffusion-weighted and dynamic contrast-enhanced MR imaging. Radiology 2010;257(3):715–23. http://dx.doi.org/10.1148/radiol.10100021.

31. Hoeks CM, Hambrock T, Yakar D, et al. Transition zone prostate cancer: detection and localization with 3-T multiparametric MR imaging. Radiology 2013;266(1):207–17. http://dx.doi.org/10.1148/radiol.12120281.

32. Noguchi M, Stamey TA, McNeal JE, et al. Relationship between systematic biopsies and histological features of 222 radical prostatectomy specimens: lack of prediction of tumor significance for men with nonpalpable prostate cancer. J Urol 2001;166(1):104–9 [discussion: 109–10].

33. deSouza NM, Reinsberg SA, Scurr ED, et al. Magnetic resonance imaging in prostate cancer: the value of apparent diffusion coefficients for identifying malignant nodules. Br J Radiol 2007;80(950):90–5. http://dx.doi.org/10.1259/bjr/24232319.

34. Tamada T, Sone T, Jo Y, et al. Apparent diffusion coefficient values in peripheral and transition zones of the prostate: comparison between normal and malignant prostatic tissues and correlation with histologic grade. J Magn Reson Imaging 2008;28(3):720–6. http://dx.doi.org/10.1002/jmri.21503.

35. Hambrock T, Somford DM, Huisman HJ, et al. Relationship between apparent diffusion coefficients at 3.0-T MR imaging and Gleason grade in peripheral zone prostate cancer. Radiology 2011. http://dx.doi.org/10.1148/radiol.091409.

36. Itou Y, Nakanishi K, Narumi Y, et al. Clinical utility of apparent diffusion coefficient (ADC) values in patients with prostate cancer: can ADC values contribute to assess the aggressiveness of prostate cancer? J Magn Reson Imaging 2011;33(1):167–72. http://dx.doi.org/10.1002/jmri.22317.

37. Turkbey B, Shah VP, Pang Y, et al. Is apparent diffusion coefficient associated with clinical risk scores for prostate cancers that are visible on 3-T MR images? Radiology 2011;258(2):488–95. http://dx.doi.org/10.1148/radiol.10100667.

38. Verma S, Rajesh A, Morales H, et al. Assessment of aggressiveness of prostate cancer: correlation of apparent diffusion coefficient with histologic grade after radical prostatectomy. AJR Am J Roentgenol 2011;196(2):374–81. http://dx.doi.org/10.2214/AJR.10.4441.

39. Kim CK, Park BK, Lee HM, et al. MRI techniques for prediction of local tumor progression after high-intensity focused ultrasonic ablation of prostate cancer. AJR Am J Roentgenol 2008;190(5):1180–6. http://dx.doi.org/10.2214/AJR.07.2924.

40. Kim CK, Park BK, Lee HM. Prediction of locally recurrent prostate cancer after radiation therapy: incremental value of 3T diffusion-weighted MRI. J Magn Reson Imaging 2009;29(2):391–7. http://dx.doi.org/10.1002/jmri.21645.

41. Park SY, Kim CK, Park BK, et al. Prediction of biochemical recurrence following radical prostatectomy in men with prostate cancer by diffusion-weighted magnetic resonance imaging: initial results. Eur Radiol 2011;21(5):1111–8. http://dx.doi.org/10.1007/s00330-010-1999-9.

42. Giannarini G, Nguyen DP, Thalmann GN, et al. Diffusion-weighted magnetic resonance imaging detects local recurrence after radical prostatectomy: initial experience. Eur Urol 2012;61(3):616–20. http://dx.doi.org/10.1016/j.eururo.2011.11.030.

43. Tekes A, Kamel I, Imam K, et al. Dynamic MRI of bladder cancer: evaluation of staging accuracy. AJR Am J Roentgenol 2005;184(1):121–7. http://dx.doi.org/10.2214/ajr.184.1.01840121.

44. Abou-El-Ghar ME, El-Assmy A, Refaie HF, et al. Bladder cancer: diagnosis with diffusion-weighted MR imaging in patients with gross hematuria. Radiology 2009;251(2):415–21. http://dx.doi.org/10.1148/radiol.2503080723.

45. Takeuchi M, Sasaki S, Ito M, et al. Urinary bladder cancer: diffusion-weighted MR imaging–accuracy for diagnosing T stage and estimating histologic grade. Radiology 2009;251(1):112–21. http://dx.doi.org/10.1148/radiol.2511080873.

46. Kobayashi S, Koga F, Yoshida S, et al. Diagnostic performance of diffusion-weighted magnetic resonance imaging in bladder cancer: potential utility of apparent diffusion coefficient values as a biomarker to predict clinical aggressiveness. Eur Radiol 2011;21(10):2178–86. http://dx.doi.org/10.1007/s00330-011-2174-7.

47. Yoshida S, Koga F, Kawakami S, et al. Initial experience of diffusion-weighted magnetic resonance imaging to assess therapeutic response to induction chemoradiotherapy against muscle-invasive bladder cancer. Urology 2010;75(2):387–91. http://dx.doi.org/10.1016/j.urology.2009.06.111.

48. Bipat S, Glas AS, Slors FJ, et al. Rectal cancer: local staging and assessment of lymph node involvement with endoluminal US, CT, and MR imaging–a meta-analysis. Radiology 2004;232(3):773–83. http://dx.doi.org/10.1148/radiol.2323031368.

49. Rao SX, Zeng MS, Chen CZ, et al. The value of diffusion-weighted imaging in combination with T2-weighted imaging for rectal cancer detection. Eur J Radiol 2008;65(2):299–303. http://dx.doi.org/10.1016/j.ejrad.2007.04.001.

50. Collette L, Bosset JF, Dulk den M, et al. Patients with curative resection of cT3-4 rectal cancer after preoperative radiotherapy or radiochemotherapy: does anybody benefit from adjuvant fluorouracil-based chemotherapy? A trial of the European Organisation for Research and Treatment of Cancer Radiation Oncology Group. J Clin Oncol 2007;25(28):4379–86. http://dx.doi.org/10.1200/JCO.2007.11.9685.

51. Das P, Skibber JM, Rodriguez-Bigas MA, et al. Clinical and pathologic predictors of locoregional recurrence, distant metastasis, and overall survival in patients treated with chemoradiation and mesorectal excision for rectal cancer. Am J Clin Oncol 2006;29(3):219–24. http://dx.doi.org/10.1097/01.coc.0000214930.78200.4a.

52. Das P, Skibber JM, Rodriguez-Bigas MA, et al. Predictors of tumor response and downstaging in patients who receive preoperative chemoradiation for rectal cancer. Cancer 2007;109(9):1750–5. http://dx.doi.org/10.1002/cncr.22625.

53. Fietkau R, Barten M, Klautke G, et al. Postoperative chemotherapy may not be necessary for patients with ypN0-category after neoadjuvant chemoradiotherapy of rectal cancer. Dis Colon Rectum 2006; 49(9):1284–92. http://dx.doi.org/10.1007/s10350-006-0570- x.

54. Park IJ, You YN, Agarwal A, et al. Neoadjuvant treatment response as an early response indicator for patients with rectal cancer. J Clin Oncol 2012; 30(15):1770–6. http://dx.doi.org/10.1200/JCO.2011.39.7901.

55. Silberfein EJ, Kattepogu KM, Hu CY, et al. Long-term survival and recurrence outcomes following surgery for distal rectal cancer. Ann Surg Oncol 2010;17(11):2863–9. http://dx.doi.org/10.1245/s10434-010-1119-8.

56. Smith KD, Tan D, Das P, et al. Clinical significance of acellular mucin in rectal adenocarcinoma patients with a pathologic complete response to preoperative chemoradiation. Ann Surg 2010;251(2): 261–4. http://dx.doi.org/10.1097/SLA.0b013e3181bdfc27.

57. Patel UB, Taylor F, Blomqvist L, et al. Magnetic resonance imaging-detected tumor response for locally advanced rectal cancer predicts survival outcomes: MERCURY experience. J Clin Oncol 2011;29(28):3753–60. http://dx.doi.org/10.1200/JCO.2011.34.9068.

58. Maretto I, Pomerri F, Pucciarelli S, et al. The potential of restaging in the prediction of pathologic response after preoperative chemoradiotherapy for rectal cancer. Ann Surg Oncol 2007;14(2):455–61. http://dx.doi.org/10.1245/s10434-006-9269-4.

59. Kuo LJ, Chern MC, Tsou MH, et al. Interpretation of magnetic resonance imaging for locally advanced rectal carcinoma after preoperative chemoradiation therapy. Dis Colon Rectum 2005;48(1):23–8.

60. Chen CC, Lee RC, Lin JK, et al. How accurate is magnetic resonance imaging in restaging rectal cancer in patients receiving preoperative combined chemoradiotherapy? Dis Colon Rectum 2005;48(4):722–8. http://dx.doi.org/10.1007/s10350-004-0851-1.

61. Kim SH, Lee JM, Hong SH, et al. Locally advanced rectal cancer: added value of diffusion-weighted MR imaging in the evaluation of tumor response to neoadjuvant chemo- and radiation therapy. Radiology 2009;253(1):116–25. http://dx.doi.org/10.1148/radiol.2532090027.

62. Sun YS, Zhang XP, Tang L, et al. Locally advanced rectal carcinoma treated with preoperative chemotherapy and radiation therapy: preliminary analysis of diffusion- weighted MR imaging for early detection of tumor histopathologic downstaging. Radiology 2010;254(1):170–8. http://dx.doi.org/10.1148/radiol.2541082230.

63. Lambregts DM, Vandecaveye V, Barbaro B, et al. Diffusion-weighted MRI for selection of complete responders after chemoradiation for locally advanced rectal cancer: a multicenter study. Ann Surg Oncol 2011;18(8):2224–31. http://dx.doi.org/10.1245/s10434-011-1607-5.

64. Song I, Kim SH, Lee SJ, et al. Value of diffusion-weighted imaging in the detection of viable tumour after neoadjuvant chemoradiation therapy in patients with locally advanced rectal cancer: comparison with T2 weighted and PET/CT imaging. Br J Radiol 2012;85(1013):577–86. http://dx.doi.org/10.1259/bjr/68424021.

65. Park MJ, Kim SH, Lee SJ, et al. Locally advanced rectal cancer: added value of diffusion-weighted MR imaging for predicting tumor clearance of the mesorectal fascia after neoadjuvant chemotherapy and radiation therapy. Radiology 2011;260(3): 771–80. http://dx.doi.org/10.1148/radiol.11102135.

66. Brændengen M, Hansson K, Radu C, et al. Delineation of gross tumor volume (GTV) for radiation

treatment planning of locally advanced rectal cancer using information from MRI or FDG-PET/CT: a prospective study. Int J Radiat Oncol Biol Phys 2011;81(4):e439–45.   http://dx.doi.org/10.1016/j.ijrobp.2011.03.031.

67. Brush J, Boyd K, Chappell F, et al. The value of FDG positron emission tomography/computerised tomography (PET/CT) in pre-operative staging of colorectal cancer: a systematic review and economic evaluation. Health Technol Assess 2011; 15(35):1–192. http://dx.doi.org/10.3310/hta15350, iii–iv.

68. Buijsen J, van den Bogaard J, Janssen MH, et al. FDG-PET provides the best correlation with the tumor specimen compared to MRI and CT in rectal cancer. Radiother Oncol 2011;98(2):270–6. http://dx.doi.org/10.1016/j.radonc.2010.11.018.

69. Jang KM, Kim SH, Choi D, et al. Pathological correlation with diffusion restriction on diffusion-weighted imaging in patients with pathological complete response after neoadjuvant chemoradiation therapy for locally advanced rectal cancer: preliminary results. Br J Radiol 2012;85(1017): e566–72. http://dx.doi.org/10.1259/bjr/24557556.

70. Masselli G, Gualdi G. MR imaging of the small bowel. Radiology 2012;264(2):333–48. http://dx.doi.org/10.1148/radiol.12111658/-/DC1.

71. Maccioni F, Patak MA, Signore A, et al. New frontiers of MRI in Crohn's disease: motility imaging, diffusion-weighted imaging, perfusion MRI, MR spectroscopy, molecular imaging, and hybrid imaging. Abdom Imaging 2012;37(6):974–82.

72. Oto A, Kayhan A, Williams JT, et al. Active Crohn's disease in the small bowel: evaluation by diffusion weighted imaging and quantitative dynamic contrast enhanced MR imaging. J Magn Reson Imaging 2011;33(3):615–24. http://dx.doi.org/10.1002/jmri.22435.

73. Oto A, Zhu F, Kulkarni K, et al. Evaluation of diffusion-weighted MR imaging for detection of bowel inflammation in patients with Crohn's disease. Acad Radiol 2009;16(5):597–603. http://dx.doi.org/10.1016/j.acra.2008.11.009.

74. Oussalah A, Laurent V, Bruot O, et al. Diffusion-weighted magnetic resonance without bowel preparation for detecting colonic inflammation in inflammatory bowel disease. Gut 2010;59(8): 1056–65. http://dx.doi.org/10.1136/gut.2009.197665.

75. Kirkham A. MRI of the penis. Br J Radiol 2012; 85(Spec No 1):S86–93. http://dx.doi.org/10.1259/bjr/63301362.

76. Tsili AC, Argyropoulou MI, Giannakis D, et al. Diffusion-weighted MR imaging of normal and abnormal scrotum: preliminary results. Asian J Androl 2012; 14(4):649–54. http://dx.doi.org/10.1038/aja.2011.172.

77. Kantarci M, Doganay S, Yalcin A, et al. Diagnostic performance of diffusion-weighted MRI in the detection of nonpalpable undescended testes: comparison with conventional MRI and surgical findings. AJR Am J Roentgenol 2010;195(4): W268–73. http://dx.doi.org/10.2214/AJR.10.4221.

78. Harisinghani MG, Barentsz J, Hahn PF, et al. Noninvasive detection of clinically occult lymph-node metastases in prostate cancer. N Engl J Med 2003;348(25):2491–9.   http://dx.doi.org/10.1056/NEJMoa022749.

79. Mizukami Y, Ueda S, Mizumoto A, et al. Diffusion-weighted magnetic resonance imaging for detecting lymph node metastasis of rectal cancer. World J Surg 2011;35(4):895–9. http://dx.doi.org/10.1007/s00268-011-0986-x.

80. Heijnen LA, Lambregts DM, Mondal D, et al. Diffusion-weighted MR imaging in primary rectal cancer staging demonstrates but does not characterise lymph nodes. Eur Radiol 2013;23(12):3354–60. http://dx.doi.org/10.1007/s00330-013-2952-5.

Magnetic Resonance Imaging in Rectal Cancer

Elizabeth Furey, MD, FRCPC*, Kartik S. Jhaveri, MD

KEYWORDS

- Rectal cancer • Preoperative staging • Magnetic resonance imaging • Rectal anatomy
- Circumferential resection margin

KEY POINTS

- Magnetic resonance (MR) imaging plays a key role in staging evaluation of rectal cancer. The cornerstone of staging MR involves high-resolution T2 imaging orthogonal to the rectal lumen.
- The goals of MR staging are identification of patients who will benefit from neoadjuvant therapy prior to surgery in order to minimize postoperative recurrence and planning of optimal surgical approach.
- MR provides excellent anatomic visualization of the rectum and mesorectal fascia (MRF), allowing for accurate prediction of circumferential resection margin (CRM) status and tumor stage.
- Improved accuracy for lymph node staging can be achieved through evaluation of node morphology, signal heterogeneity, and dynamic enhancement characteristics in addition to size.
- MR has an evolving role for the evaluation of neoadjuvant treatment response, further triaging optimal patient treatment and surgical approach.

INTRODUCTION

Rectal cancer is one of the most common malignancies, with an incidence of 40 in 100,000.[1] Colorectal cancer is the third leading cause of cancer-related mortality worldwide in both men and women.[2] In 2013, an estimated 140,000 new colorectal malignancies will be diagnosed in the United States alone, and more than one-quarter of these will arise from the rectum.[2] Rectal cancers are associated with poorer prognosis and higher local recurrence than their counterparts in the colon. Although precise staging of rectal cancer is possible only with a surgical specimen, progress in preoperative management has necessitated the advent of accurate staging methods prior to surgical resection. Total mesorectal excision (TME) is the standard of care, with additional neoadjuvant concurrent chemoradiation therapy (CCRT) in a select group of patients. In patients with advanced local-stage disease, neoadjuvant CCRT has improved local control and is associated with reduced toxicity when compared with postoperative adjuvant therapy.[3] As such, initial staging investigations should identify the patients who benefit from preoperative therapy with intent to minimize the risk of tumor recurrence, while avoiding unnecessary treatment of patients in whom no benefit has been shown. Preoperative staging can also assist in surgical planning, identifying candidates for sphincter-preserving surgery. In this regard, high spatial resolution MR imaging has been established as an accurate preoperative staging technique and plays a critical role in pretreatment staging and evaluation for recurrence. In more recent years, the role of MR imaging has expanded to include evaluation of neoadjuvant therapy response, further tailoring surgical approaches and oncologic treatment options. MR restaging is of particular utility at institutions that

Abdominal Imaging, University Health Network, Mount Sinai and Women's College Hospital, 610 University Avenue, 3-957, Toronto, ON M5G 2M9, Canada
* Corresponding author.
E-mail address: beth.a.furey@gmail.com

Magn Reson Imaging Clin N Am 22 (2014) 165–190
http://dx.doi.org/10.1016/j.mric.2014.01.004
1064-9689/14/$ – see front matter © 2014 Elsevier Inc. All rights reserved.

have adopted organ-preserving techniques, such as transanal excision and nonoperative management (ie, a wait-and-see approach) for clinical CR.

CURRENT CONCEPTS IN RECTAL CANCER

Surgical resection is the mainstay of curative therapy for rectal cancer. TME is the standard of care, which involves radical removal of the entire rectal compartment with surrounding mesorectum through identification of naturally occurring tissue planes of the MRF.[4] The risk of local recurrence is considerably lower when the rectum is excised intact.[5] For tumors in the high rectum, low anterior resection (LAR) is the surgery of choice, whereby a portion of the distal rectum can be preserved. Tumors in the mid- to low-rectum are resected to the level of the pelvic floor muscles. For more distal tumors, sphincter-sparing surgeries, such as ultra-LAR with coloanal anastomosis and intersphincteric resection with coloanal anastomosis, may be attempted. Utilization of a sphincter-sparing technique results in improved surgical outcome in terms of recurrence and postoperative leak[6] and substantially improves quality of life in postoperative patients. Abdominoperineal resection (APR) includes removal of the entire sphincter complex and is reserved for tumors in the low rectum that are fixed to adjacent pelvic organs or structures.[7] Patients with operable locally advanced tumor or recurrent tumors are considered for total pelvic exenteration, which involves complete resection of the pelvic viscera and draining lymphatics, with the objective of removing all malignant disease.

The CRM is a pathologic term that refers to the surgically dissected surface of the specimen and corresponds to the nonperitonealized portion of the rectum.[8] A negative CRM is defined as greater than or equal to 1 mm between the tumor edge and the surgical margin and is associated with a significantly lower risk of local recurrence than a positive CRM (<1 mm).[9] The relationship of tumor to the anterior peritoneal reflection is important when considering CRM, because the anterior peritoneal reflection extends in a nearly circumferential fashion around the upper rectum but only involves the anterior aspect of the lower rectum (**Fig. 1**). The term, CRM, is not appropriate for tumors involving the upper and/or anterior peritonealized portion of the rectum.

The MRF is the extraperitoneal pelvic fascial plane that surrounds the mesorectum. CRM is defined by the surgical specimen, the goal of which is to approximate MRF. MRF is visualized on MR imaging and is a more appropriate term for MR reporting. As with CRM, the term MRF only applies to nonperitonealized portion of the rectum.

IMAGING MODALITIES IN RECTAL CANCER DIAGNOSIS AND STAGING

MR imaging is the primary imaging modality for local staging evaluation for rectal cancer. Compared with other cross-sectional imaging modalities, the main benefits of MR imaging include high soft tissue contrast resolution for tumor delineation and ability to visualize and assess MRF/CRM and its relationship to the tumor and evaluation of regional lymph nodes. MR has an established role in initial staging but in more recent years utilization has evolved to include evaluation of treatment response and local recurrence.

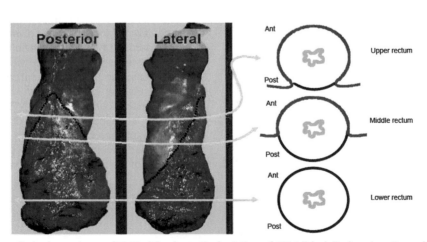

Fig. 1. Gross pathologic specimen of TME with schematic depiction of CRM (*black line*) and peritonealized rectum (*red line*). The anterior aspect of the upper rectum is predominantly peritonealized, whereas the lower rectum is entirely nonperitonealized. Ant, anterior; Post, posterior. (*Courtesy of* Dr Mahmoud Khalifa, Toronto, ON.)

Endorectal ultrasound (EUS) is an accurate method for evaluating involvement of mural invasion in early-stage rectal adenocarcinoma and in some institutions is used in staging of rectal cancer. Although EUS is accurate for staging superficial rectal tumors, it has limited utility in the staging of more advanced disease, because the depth of acoustic penetration is generally unable to assess advanced-stage disease.[10] In a prospective study by Fernandez-Esparrach and colleagues,[11] T staging accuracy for EUS was similar to MR imaging for T2 and T3 tumors. MR imaging did not visualize any T1 tumor, and EUS understaged all T4 tumors. Accuracy of MR for nodal staging is higher than EUS.[12] EUS also tends to overstage T2 tumors. In a randomized controlled trial by Sauer and colleagues,[3] 20% of tumors staged as T3 or T4 by EUS were pathologically staged as T2. Additional limitations include operator dependence, patient tolerance, probe limitations, and inability to examine proximal to obstructing tumors. Hence, EUS has a high accuracy in the evaluation of early-stage tumors but is less suitable than MR imaging for the evaluation of the mesorectal excision plane or evaluation of mesorectal and extra-mesorectal lymph nodes.[13]

CT is not recommended for local staging of rectal cancer, because it cannot reliably differentiate layers of the rectal wall, identify the MRF, or depict tumor invasion in surrounding pelvic structures.[14] In evaluation of the MRF, multidetector-row CT does not correlate well enough with MR imaging findings to replace it in rectal cancer staging.[15] CT is essentially used to assess distant metastatic disease, such as liver and lung metastases.

MR IMAGING TECHNIQUE

MR technique is somewhat variable according to institution, but the universal goal of MR imaging is acquisition of high-resolution T2-weighted images with small field of view (FOV) thin-section imaging for evaluation of the primary tumor and its relationship to pelvic structures[16] as well as assessment regional lymph nodes.

Prior to an MR imaging examination, obtaining clinical information assists in planning the MR scan, including tumor location, circumferential extent, and distance from anal verge.[17] The examination may take up 45 minutes, so patients should be positioned comfortably in a supine position. In general, no bowel preparation is required. An empty bladder is preferable. Use of an antispasmodic agent (ie, glucagon or buscopan) helps eliminate bowel motion artifact and is used at the authors' institution in the absence of contraindications. In patients who cannot tolerate the length of an examination, obtaining a high-resolution T2 sequence is critical, and the protocol may be modified to accomplish this by shortening or omission of other T2 sequences. Use of gel or luminal contrast in staging of primary rectal cancer is controversial. Distending the rectum with gel may alter the distance from MRF or the sphincter complex, and instillation of gel may stimulate rectal sphincter contraction, potentially resulting in motion artifact. Some studies suggest benefit, however, in staging of smaller or polypoid tumors or in patients who have had prior radiation. Gel can also help identify the location of attachment to the rectal wall. If rectal gel or luminal contrast is considered, no more than 60 to 100 cm^3 is recommended.[18] In the authors' practice, rectal MR imaging is performed without utilization of rectal gel or luminal contrast.

Phased-array body/pelvis coils provide better signal, greater coverage, and more homogeneity than endorectal (surface) coils. The coil should be positioned to cover rectum, mesorectum, and highest nodal drainage bin, approximately 5 cm superior to the tumor. In general, this provides coverage from sacral promontory to below pubic symphysis. The lower edge of coil should be 10 cm below the pubic symphysis to acquire adequate signal from the low rectum and anus.[17] A 3.0-T system can provide faster image acquisition and improved signal-to-noise ratio. 3-D acquisitions may be possible, which can simplify the examination by removing the need for acquisition of additional 2-D image sequences in different planes. 3-D acquisitions have been shown to have comparable accuracy to 1.5-T 2-D image acquisitions.[19] In the authors' experience, 3-T imaging provides increased signal-to-noise ratio in obtaining high-resolution images, which has been substantiated in the evaluation of other pelvic tumors.[20] Imaging parameters should be adjusted accordingly for 1.5-T or 3-T systems.

Endorectal coils provide high-resolution images that are able to delineate bowel wall layers.[21] Some investigators have reported superior diagnostic accuracy compared with phased-array coils alone for T staging, with sensitivity reaching 100% and specificity of 86%.[22] As with endorectal ultrasound, there are several drawbacks of a primary endorectal MR imaging technique as well as increased cost and examination time. Developments in MR imaging phased-array coil technology have enabled high spatial resolution, high-contrast resolution scanning, which provides information comparable to that obtained with an endorectal coil.[23] Endorectal coils are thus not used routinely in practice for rectal cancer staging.

The mainstay of MR evaluation for rectal cancer is T2 fast spin-echo imaging. An initial sagittal localizer sequence should be obtained from sidewall to sidewall, which identifies the primary tumor. This sequence is also used for planning high-resolution T2 axial images orthogonal to the rectum involved by tumor. Subsequently, large FOV axial and coronal T2 sequences of the entire pelvis should be obtained. Involvement of the peritoneal reflection and pelvic sidewalls is most clearly depicted on sagittal and coronal images. Triplanar imaging is of particular utility in the assessment of large or tortuous tumors where positioning of a single axial plane is difficult. Suzuki and colleagues[24] have found that using a protocol, including triplanar T2 sequences with high-resolution imaging, resulted in significantly better correlation with histopathology regarding anterior organ involvement (sensitivity 86 vs 50% and specificity 94 vs 33%).

High-resolution T2 thin-section sequence with smaller FOV of 16 to 20 cm and slice thickness of 3 mm should be obtained through the primary tumor. Proper planning of high-resolution T2 imaging sequences is essential to staging accuracy.[25] The initial sagittal sequence is used for planning of the orthogonal plane T2 high-resolution images. Determining the site of tumor origin from the rectal wall allows for correct positioning, the orthogonal plane. This sequence must be perpendicular to long axis of rectum at the level of tumor because it provides the most accurate evaluation of tumor, depth of mural or transmural invasion, and distance from the CRM, as shown in **Fig. 2**. Obtaining images not perpendicular to the axis of tumor may result in misinterpretation due to volume averaging; for example, blurring of muscularis propria or pseudospiculated appearance that could lead to overstaging.[18] In bulky tumors or if there is tortuosity of the colon, it may be necessary to obtain images at multiple angles.

In patients with low rectal cancers, high spatial resolution coronal oblique T2 through the sphincter complex depicts the relationship of the tumor to the rectal wall. This sequence provides information on intersphincteric plane and levator muscle involvement.

Conventional T1 images are not helpful for bowel wall layer depiction, because of similar relaxation rates of bowel wall and tumor. T1 imaging primarily provides information about pelvic bones and, in some cases, nodal anatomy.

The addition of diffusion-weighted images (DWIs) to T2-weighted images improves accuracy for rectal cancer detection.[26,27] Images are acquired in the axial plane with the patient in free breathing, from the level of the aortic bifurcation to the upper thigh, in order to include *inferior mesenteric* lymph nodes and groin nodes. In the authors' practice, diffusion gradients at 4 time points (or b values) are obtained (b values 0, 50, 400, and 800). An apparent diffusion coefficient (ADC) map is subsequently generated using all b values. Low b-value images (0 and 50) provide maximal lesion detection, particularly for the presence of lymph nodes and bone metastases, whereas high b-value images (b value 800) provide signal suppression of highly cellular structures, such as gastrointestinal and urogenital lining, to maximize conspicuity of tumor.[28] The high signal

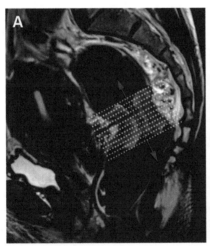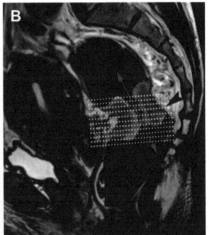

Fig. 2. Sagittal T2-weighted image used for planning high-resolution T2 sequence. (*A*) Plane of planned images (*white dotted lines*) is perpendicular to the axis of rectum/tumor (*red arrow* [*A, B*]). Incorrect selection of imaging plane (*B*) results in poor delineation of muscular layer due to averaging through a plane oblique to the tumor and rectum (*arrowhead* [*B*]).

intensity focus depicting a tissue with restricted diffusion is readily apparent against a low signal intensity background of bowel wall and feces on high b-value images. Hence, the sequence generally aids in detection of small tumors not seen on T2 images.

DWI has several limitations. Accuracies for tumor detection have been reported up to 90%,[26,27] but benign tumors may show restricted diffusion. Also, the lower spatial resolution of DWI sequences may make it more difficult to detect small lesions. False-positive results may result from air-filled colon and from slice thickness in small tumors. Hyperintensity due to collapsed bowel wall may also mimic disease. For this reason, it has been suggested that evaluation of ADC may be more reliable, although some investigators think that ADC evaluation is cumbersome in practice.

DWI is highly sensitive in nodal detection but has limited value for characterizing lymph nodes, because there is significant overlap in ADC values for benign and malignant nodes. A recent study performed by Mizukami and colleagues[29] comparing DWI and conventional MR assessment to histopathologic specimen found that the node based sensitivity is 97% and negative predictive value 84%, whereas specificity was much lower (81%), resulting in a positive predictive value of only 52%.

Gadolinium contrast has not proved effective for rectal cancer staging. Jao and colleagues[30] have found that gadolinium-enhanced T1-weighted MR imaging does not increase the diagnostic yield for tumor and nodal staging and can be omitted from the staging protocol. It has also been shown that contrast enhancement does not improve diagnostic accuracy for assessment of tumor penetration through rectal wall and tumor extension into MRF.[31] Dynamic imaging is used, however, as part of the authors' routine multiparametric protocol to increase confidence levels for detection of small tumors, characterizing nodes, assessing treatment response, and evaluating any incidental pelvic or bone abnormalities detected during the examination (Table 1).

RELEVANT ANATOMY

Anatomic landmarks important to rectal cancer surgery may be defined on MR imaging, which is of use in staging tumors, assessing resectability, planning surgery, and selecting patients for preoperative neoadjuvant therapy.[32]

The anal verge is an important surgical landmark, because it is easily identified at physical examination. It marks the most distal aspect of the anal canal. The location of the lower border

of the tumor should be determined relative to this line, which is most easily depicted on sagittal images (Fig. 3).

The anal canal comprises an internal sphincter and external sphincter complex, separated by a thin, fat-containing intersphincteric plane (Fig. 4). The internal sphincter is a continuation of the smooth muscle layer of the rectum. The external sphincter complex begins cranially at the inferior insertion of levator ani muscles and includes the puborectalis muscle and the more inferior external sphincter muscles,[18] shown in Fig. 4. The anatomic relationship of the most inferior aspect of the tumor for the top border of the anal sphincter (ie, puborectalis) and the depth of involvement of tumor is of critical importance in MR imaging evaluation, because it identifies patients who may not be candidates for sphincter preservation surgery.

Identification of rectal wall layers allows for accurate T staging. The outer muscular layer is readily apparent by MR imaging as a hypointense line. The inner mucosa and submucosa are indistinguishable as a thicker band of slightly higher signal intensity. Perirectal fat is identified as high signal intensity surrounding the outer muscular layer.

The anterior peritoneal reflection separates the intra- and extraperitoneal portions of the rectum and is a well-defined anatomic landmark at laparotomy.[33] Experienced radiologists identify the anterior peritoneal relection in more than 80% of cases.[34] In the midsagittal plane, the anterior peritoneal reflection consisted of a thin T2 hypointense line 1 mm or less in thickness on most MR imaging studies (Fig. 6). The peritoneum extends over the surface of the bladder posteriorly to the point of attachment at the junction of the upper two-thirds and lower one-third of the rectum. In men, the tip of the seminal vesicles is a consistent landmark for the location of the most inferior portion of the peritoneal membrane. In women, the location is variable, but the reflection is commonly seen at the uterocervical angle. A trace amount of fluid in the pelvic cul-de-sac increases the conspicuity of the anterior peritoneal reflection.[34] The peritoneum attaches in a V-shaped manner onto the anterior aspect of the rectum (Fig. 5), an appearance characterized by Brown and colleagues[32] as the seagull sign. The peritoneum-lined recess between the rectum and the posterior aspect of the bladder is termed, the rectovesical pouch. Proper assessment of the anterior peritoneal reflection requires evaluation of both axial and sagittal images.[35] The ability to visualize the anterior peritoneal reflection and its relationship with rectal tumor on MR imaging has implications for

Table 1
MR imaging parameters

	MR Imaging Sequence					
	Sagittal T2 FSE	Axial T2 FSE	Coronal T2 FSE	Oblique Hi-res T2 FSE	DWI	T1 FSPGR
Repetition time (ms)	3500	3320	3500	4000	5800	4.44
Echo time (ms)	91	91	91	80	96	1.59
Number of slices	28	40	25	15	30	32
Bandwidth (Hz/Px)	391	391	391	391	1132	400
FOV (mm)	220	220	220	200	250	240
Slice thickness (mm)	3	4	4	3	4	4
Distance factor (%)	25	25	25	0	20	20
Phase FOV (%)	100	100	100	100	100	100
Number of acquisitions	3	2	2	3	6	1
Matrix	350 × 263	350 × 263	350 × 263	350 × 263	250 × 250	240 × 240
Phase encode direction	Anterioposterior	Transverse (R>L)	Transverse (R>L)	Anterioposterior	Anterioposterior	Anterioposterior
Saturation band	Anterior	N/A	N/A	Superior and inferior	N/A	N/A
Acquisition time (minutes)	4	5.5	4	5	4.5	1
Base resolution	320	320	320	320	192	320
Voxel size (mm)	0.7 × 0.7 × 4.0	0.7 × 0.7 × 4.0	0.7 × 0.7 × 4.0	0.6 × 0.6 × 3.0	1.7 × 1.3 × 4.0	0.9 × 0.8 × 4.0

Abbreviations: FSE, fast spin echo; FSPGR, fast spoiled gradient echo; Hi-res, high resolution; L, left; N/A, not applicable; Px, pixel; R, right.

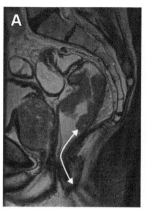
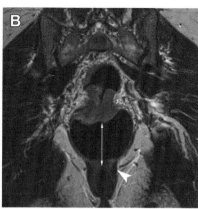

Fig. 3. (A) Sagittal image demonstrating distance from anal verge to the most inferior aspect of the tumor (*arrow*). (B) Coronal image in a different patient demonstrates distance from the top of the anal sphincter complex to the most inferior aspect of the tumor (*arrow*). The top of the sphincter complex is demarcated by the puborectalis (*arrowhead*).

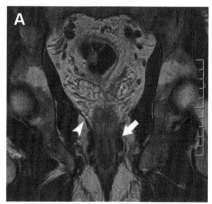
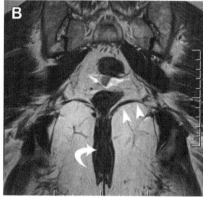

Fig. 4. Coronal images in 2 different patients show internal anal sphincter as a smooth continuation of the rectum. (A) Puborectalis is depicted as part of the external anal sphincter complex (*solid arrow [A]*). (B) Levator ani (*arrowheads [A, B]*) and intersphincteric plane (*curved arrow [B]*).

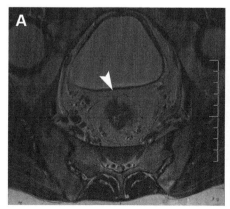
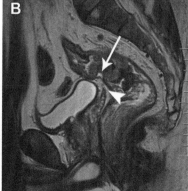

Fig. 5. Axial (A) and sagittal (B) T2-weighted images of anterior peritoneal reflection. (A) Note the V-shaped attachment of the peritoneum onto the anterior aspect of the rectum, known as the seagull sign (*arrowhead*). (B) In the sagittal plane, the attachment is seen as a thin hypointense line (*arrow*) at the tip of the seminal vesicles (*arrowhead*).

spread of tumor and allows for further individualization of treatment.

MRF is consistently visualized on MR imaging as a distinct thin T2 hypointense layer surrounding the mesorectum and is best seen on axial images (see **Fig. 6**). It is difficult to recognize the MRF at the distal and anterior portions of the rectum because of the small amount of fat tissue.[36]

The rectoprostatic fascia, or Denonvilliers fascia, is a focal thickening of the MRF at midline anteriorly that separates the prostate and urinary bladder from the rectum. It is a single fibromuscular structure that contains several fused layers (**Fig. 7**).

IMAGING FINDINGS
T Staging

Goals of preoperative imaging in rectal cancer include accurate tumor localization, sphincter involvement, depth of mural involvement and extramural extension into mesorectal fat, evaluation of MRF for threatened resection margin, status of peritoneal reflection, and identification of extramural vascular invasion (EMVI) and nodal metastases (**Table 2**).

For purposes of MR reporting, the rectum is divided longitudinally into thirds (**Fig. 8**). A tumor is located in the upper third of the rectum if it is more than 10 cm from the anal verge. Because tumors at this level are generally covered anteriorly by the anterior peritoneal reflection, the relationship to the peritoneal reflection (eg, above, straddles, or below) at this level is important. A tumor arising in the midthird of the rectum is between 5

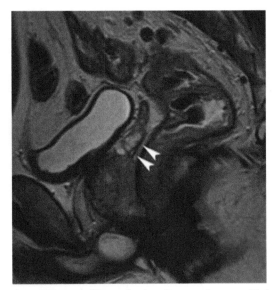

Fig. 7. Denonvilliers fascia. Paramedian sagittal T2-weighted image demonstrates a thin hypointense line posterior to the caudal portion of the seminal vesicles (*arrowheads*).

and 10 cm from the anal verge, where the rectum is usually encircled by mesorectal fat. A tumor is located in the lower third if it is less than 5 cm from the anal verge. Tumors residing here may be at or below the sphincter complex, requiring special considerations for MR reporting. Craniocaudal location of rectal tumor is frequently significant for surgical planning. Patients with tumors in the mid- and high-rectum are usually candidates for sphincter-sparing surgery, whereas patients with low rectal tumors have variable candidacy for sphincter preservation.

Thin-section, high-resolution T2 images in a plane perpendicular to the axis of the involved rectum are highly accurate for evaluation of tumor extent.[37,38] Tumor demonstrates intermediate T2 intensity, distinct from the hyperintense submucosal layer and hypointense muscular layer (**Fig. 9**).

T1 Lesions

T1 lesions confined to submucosa are seen at MR imaging as hypointense to the surrounding submucosa. Because there is no penetration to the muscular layer, a discrete intact hyperintense ring of submucosa deep to the deep margin of the tumor may be visible. The intact submucosal layer is variably present and visualization is not necessary for the diagnosis of a T1 tumor. T1 tumors may be difficult to accurately stage with MR imaging, and phased array coil MR imaging may not reliably differentiate T1 and T2 tumors.

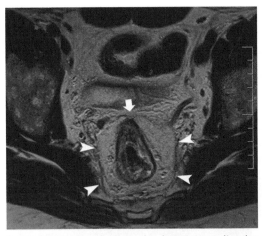

Fig. 6. MRF is identified as a thin hypointense line (*arrowheads*) surrounding the mesorectal fat. Note the peritoneal attachment to the rectum at its anterior aspect, delineating the anterior peritoneal reflection (*arrow*).

		TNM Staging of Rectal Cancer
Table 2		
TNM staging of rectal cancer with MR imaging		
T stage	Tx	Primary tumor cannot be assessed
	T0	No evidence of primary tumor
	Tis	Carcinoma in situ
	T1	Tumor invades submucosa
	T2	Tumor invades muscularis propria
	T3	Tumor invades through muscularis propria to pericolorectal tissues
	a	Tumor <5 mm into the perirectal fat or extramural
	b	Tumor 5–10 mm into the perirectal fat or extramural
	c	Tumor >10 mm into the perirectal fat or extramural
	T4	Organ invasion
	a	Tumor penetrates to surface of visceral peritoneum
	b	Tumor directly invades or is adherent to other organs or structures
N stage	Nx	Regional lymph nodes cannot be assessed
	N0	No regional lymph node metastasis
	N1	Metastasis in 1–3 regional lymph nodes
	N2 a	Metastasis in one regional lymph node
	b	Metastasis in 2–3 regional lymph nodes
M stage	M0	No distant metastais
	M1 a	Metastasis confined to one organ or site
	b	Metastasis in more than one organ or site or peritoneum

Adapted from Edge S, Byrd DR, Compton CC, et al (eds.). AJCC Cancer Staging Manual. 7th ed. New York: Springer, 2010. p. 143–64; and Hussain S, et al (July 2012). MR Rectum Cancer. In Langlotz CP (ed.): RSNA rectal MRI reporting template. Retrieved from http://www.radreport.org/template/0000068.

T2 Lesions

T2 lesions extend into the hypointense muscularis propria layer, without breaching the outer margin. At MR imaging, tumor is seen as intermediate signal (higher than muscle and lower than submucosa) that does not extend beyond the outer margin of the muscular layer (see **Fig. 9**).

T3 Lesions

T3 tumors are transmural in extent and involve mesorectal fat but do not involve the serosal

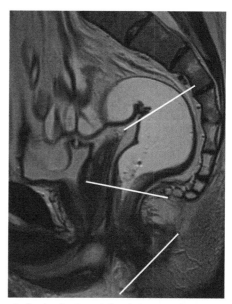

Fig. 8. Sagittal T2-weighted image depicting the approximate location of the upper-, mid-, and low-rectum (*white lines*). The most inferior line is coincident with the anal verge, defined as the inferiormost aspect of the anal sphincter complex.

surfaces or invade adjacent structures. In general, the extension beyond the muscular layer has a broad-based nodular configuration within the perirectal fat. Continuity of tumor signal in perirectal fat with the intramural portion of the tumor is crucial. Disruption in the outer muscular layer does not necessitate tumor invasion, because small

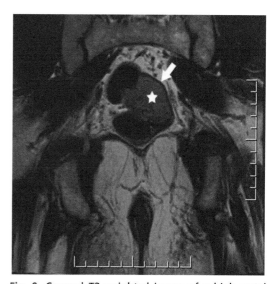

Fig. 9. Coronal T2-weighted image of a high rectal tumor demonstrating intermediate tumor signal intensity (*star*) as well as the intact hypointense muscular layer (*arrow*).

penetrating wall vessels may give this appearance.[39] Thin spiculations may also represent peritumoral fibrosis and are not sensitive or specific in the diagnosis of T3 lesions.[40] Tumoral nodules within mesorectal fat separate from the tumor itself are also considered as T3 stage.[41]

T2 Versus Early T3 Lesions

The ability to distinguish T2 from early T3 lesions lies in the distinction of spiculation of perirectal fat due to peritumoral fibrosis from fibrosis with tumor infiltration.[42] MR imaging does not differentiate well between T2 and early T3 lesions, but this distinction is unlikely to be of clinical significance because patients with early T3 lesions receive little benefit from preoperative neoadjuvant therapy.[16] In tumors where there is spiculation of the mesorectal fat, making assessment difficult, reporting tumor as T2/early T3 allows the multidisciplinary team to tailor therapy in the overall assessment of the patient (**Figs. 10 and 11**).

Extramural Depth of Invasion

Although depth of invasion beyond muscularis propria is not considered in TMN staging, it has been shown in several studies to confer considerable prognostic importance. The extent of extramural disease involvement in tumors that are clearly T3 is an independent prognostic factor,[43,44] and the distance of tumor involvement from the CRM is a more robust predictor of local recurrence than T stage.[45,46] A universal goal of neoadjuvant CCRT is to decrease tumor bulk to provide clear

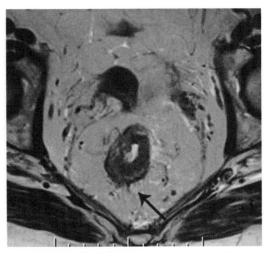

Fig. 11. Peritumoral fibrosis. Axial T2-weighted image shows spiculation of mesorectal fat at the 6-o'clock position (*arrow*) suggestive of peritumoral desmoplastic reaction. This renders distinction between T2 and early T3 difficult. Note that no nodular tumoral components extend beyond the muscular layer. Pathology at the time of TME revealed T2 tumor.

surgical margins at the time of resection, performing surgery with curative intent. In this regard, it is important to identify tumors that involve the MRF or threaten positive margins at the time of surgical excision. Merkel and colleagues[45] have shown that T3 tumors with greater than 5 mm of extramural invasion have cancer related 5-year survival of only 54%, whereas T3 tumors with less than 5 mm of extramural invasion have disease-specific 5-year survival of 85% when treatment consists of surgery alone. Hence, patients with early T3 tumors have similar prognosis to T1 and T2 tumors, and little benefit from preoperative adjuvant CCRT is conferred to a patient with T1, T2, or early T3 tumor.[47] These findings were reiterated by the Magnetic Resonance Imaging and Rectal Cancer European Equivalence (MERCURY) multi-institutional study, which also affirmed the accuracy of high-resolution MR imaging in estimating depth of tumor invasion from CRM within 0.5 mm of measurement of the histopathologic specimen.[25] Therefore, it is important not only to report an accurate T stage but also to stratify good and poor prognostic T3 lesions, which can be achieved by determining the depth of extramural involvement beyond muscularis propria (**Fig. 12**). The Radiological society of North America's reporting template (www.radreport.org/txt/00000068) includes stratification of T3 tumors into stage T3a through T3c. This is considered an optional stratification by American Joint Committee on Cancer.[41]

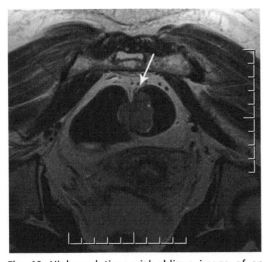

Fig. 10. High-resolution axial oblique image of an early-stage polypoid lesion. Intact low signal intensity layer (*arrow*) is identified circumferentially throughout the distended rectum.

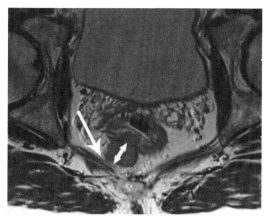

Fig. 12. Depth of extramural invasion. High-resolution axial oblique T2 images depicting a low rectal tumor, which has a large nodular extension beyond the muscularis propria (*double arrow*), compatible with an advanced stage T3 lesion. The MRF is not well seen due to the inferior location of the tumor, but the close proximity to the levator musculature (*arrow*) presumes a threatened margin.

T4 Lesions

Due to the ability of high-resolution MR imaging to visualize the anterior peritoneal reflection, the latest TNM classification differentiates tumor violation of the peritoneal reflection (T4a) from invasion into other pelvic structures (T4b) **(Figs. 13 and 14)**.[48] T4 lesions at the anterior aspect of the rectum may involve urinary bladder, prostate, and uterus. Lateral and posterior tumors may involve pelvic sidewalls or sacrum. Threatened

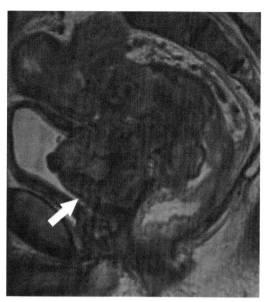

Fig. 14. Stage T4b tumor. Sagittal T2-weighted image demonstrates a large T4b lesion invading the posterior wall of the urinary bladder. Tumor invades through bladder mucosa and is seen within the bladder lumen (*arrow*).

anterior peritoneal reflection margin usually necessitates preoperative CCRT. Involvement of the sidewall also alters the surgical approach and necessitates preoperative neoadjuvant therapy **(Table 3)**.

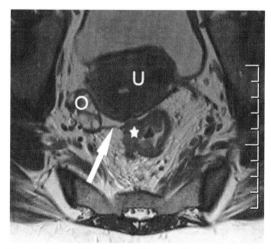

Fig. 13. Stage T4a tumor. High-resolution axial oblique image depicting a nodular tumor component outside the bowel lumen (*star*) with invasion of the anterior peritoneal reflection (*arrow*). O, right ovary; U, uterus.

Table 3 T staging with MR imaging	
MR Imaging T Staging	
T1 or T2	No breech of T2 hypointense line representing muscularis propria
T2 or early T3	Spiculation of perirectal fat
T3	Broad or nodular base of tumor extending beyond muscularis propria Include depth of extramural invasion for T3 subcategorization
T4	Abnormal signal intensity invades peritoneal reflection (T4a) or other organs/pelvic sidewall (T4b)

Adapted from Al-Sukhni E, Milot L, Fruitman M, et al. User's Guide for the Synoptic MRI Report for Rectal Cancer. In: MacDonald B, Jhaveri J, Gill D, editors. Cancer Care Ontario. Retrieved from https://www.cancercare.on.ca/toolbox/SoPTools/sop_qi_resources/colorectal/.

The relationship of the tumor to the MRF is crucial for surgical planning and can reliably be assessed with MR imaging. The shortest distance should be regarded as the closest distance from either tumor margin, tumoral deposit or lymph node, or vascular invasion (ie, tumor thrombus). Due to the lack of sensitivity and specificity of peritumoral spiculation in the mesorectal fat, it is advisable to report the distance from the spiculation to CRM and most penetrating part of tumor to CRM separately. There is some controversy regarding distance of tumor from the MRF that predicts a safe surgical margin at the MRF. Beets-Tan and colleagues[42] have determined that a tumor-free margin of 1 mm is predictable when the distance from tumor to MRF is 5 mm or greater. This is in contradistinction to an early study by Brown and colleagues,[16] wherein the distance from tumor to MRF as measured on MR imaging was determined to be equivalent to histopathology. Similar findings were later emphasized by the MERCURY study group.[23] Notwithstanding, both groups have demonstrated MR imaging to be a highly accurate tool in the assessment of extramural depth of invasion and involvement of MRF on final histopathology. A more recent study has found increasing the definition of a positive margin from measurements of 1 or 2 mm to 5 mm has no difference in the rate of positive resection margin or tumor recurrence and that 1 mm is a safe distance to predict negative margin (**Figs. 15** and **16**). Using a margin greater than 1 mm may result in unnecessary neoadjuvant therapy.[49]

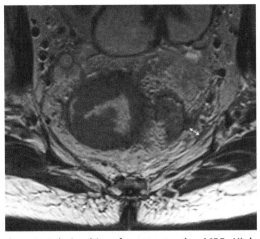

Fig. 15. Relationship of tumor to the MRF. High-resolution axial oblique image of a T3 lesion with large left satellite nodule in the 3-o'clock position. The closest distance to the MRF (*double-headed arrow*) should be measured from the closer of either tumor or satellite nodule.

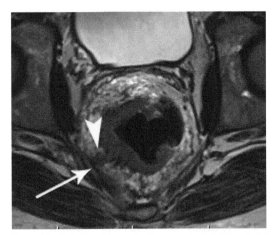

Fig. 16. Relationship of tumor to MRF. Axial T2-weighted image demonstrating an advanced stage T3 lesion with satellite tumoral nodule at the 8-o'clock position (*arrowhead*) contacting the MRF (*arrow*), implying positive CRM.

Uncommonly, a component of the tumor other than the most penetrating part is closest to the MRF. This is most likely to occur with anterior tumors involving the peritoneal reflection where there is T3 tumor above the peritoneal reflection but only T2 tumor below the peritoneal reflection. In these cases, it is important to comment on the distance from MRF of the T2 component, because it may require neoadjuvant chemoradiation if the surgical margin is threatened.

EMVI refers to invasion of large vessels deep to the muscular layer. EMVI is not included in staging but has prognostic significance. Venous invasion has been shown to be the third strongest predictor of metastatic disease.[50] MR assessment of EMVI is moderately sensitive (62%) and highly specific (88%).[51] Small vessels may be difficult to assess but involvement of larger vessels (eg, superior rectal artery or vein) is suggested by visualization of intraluminal tumor. EMVI on MR imaging should be called present when there is obvious irregularity of a vessel or intermediate intraluminal signal in vessels close to tumor replacing flow voids (**Fig. 17**). Focal expansion of the vessel lumen may be apparent. EMVI is absent when there is no tumor extension in close proximity to vascular structure; pattern of tumor invasion through muscularis propria is not nodular. If there is stranding near a vessel, EMVI is considered absent if the vessels are normal in caliber and signal intensity.[40,51]

N Staging

Mesorectal lymph nodes constitute the initial nodal drainage of rectal tumors,[52] followed by

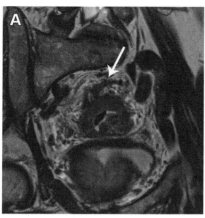
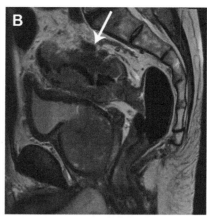

Fig. 17. EMVI. High-resolution T2-weighted coronal oblique (*A*) and sagittal (*B*) images of large high-rectal T3 lesion with EMVI. There is focal expansion of a small perirectal vessel with intermediate intraluminal signal (*arrows*, [*A, B*]).

superior rectal and inferior mesenteric vessels. Extramesorectal nodes are most commonly found along the middle rectal artery, the internal iliac chain, obturator, median sacral, and, less commonly, external or common iliac nodes.[53] Inguinal nodes represent a nonregional site of nodal metastasis and are more commonly identified in low rectal cancers. Inguinal nodes are associated with a poor prognosis and have a high association with diffuse disease.[54]

By TMN staging, N1 is defined by 1 to 3 positive regional lymph nodes, and N2 is defined by 4 or more positive nodes.[41] Assessment of mesorectal nodes is important for surgical planning so that surgeons can stay clear of these nodes during TME, although they should be completely excised. Additionally, the presence of involved lateral nodes at the pelvic sidewall is significant in terms of prognosis and treatment planning. Patients with involved pelvic sidewall nodes may undergo extended-field neoadjuvant RT, so individual extramesorectal nodes merit comment at initial staging MR imaging. Involvement of pelvic sidewall nodes may be a predictor of decreased overall survival and local recurrence.[55]

MR imaging evaluation of lymph nodes is challenging and has been a topic of extensive research. Lymph node size has been shown a poor predictor in the determination of malignancy, because disease is commonly present in nodes less than 5 mm.[56] One large series determined that all metastatic nodes are 5 mm or less in up to 30% of patients.[57] Brown and colleagues[58] have shown that no particular size cutoff is useful in predicting nodal status, because 15% of involved lymph nodes are less than 5 mm. In several studies, however, lymph nodes greater than 8 mm were highly specific for metastatic

involvement, and this has been accepted as a predictor of nodal status based on size alone.[58–60] This cutoff value for size compromises sensitivity for specificity. Assessment of border contour and signal intensity characteristics is the most accurate in assessment for disease involvement (**Fig. 18**). Using the criterion of mixed signal intensity results in high specificity and low sensitivity but combined with evaluation of nodal border contour yields much higher sensitivity and accuracy, because virtually all reactive nodes have uniform signal intensity and sharply demarcated borders. For lateral pelvic lymph nodes in particular, an ovoid shape with transverse diameter of 5 mm or greater has been suggested as the optimal criteria for lymph node metastasis,[60] although this is currently not widely used as a diagnostic criteria. Most malignant lymph nodes are found at the level of the tumor or within 5 cm proximal of the tumor.[61] Intuitively, this correlates with nodal drainage patterns of the rectum.

DWI is a useful adjunct to conventional T2 imaging, increasing the sensitivity of small lymph nodes. Recently, a study by Mir and colleagues[62] has shown that DWI detects a significant number of subcentimeter lymph nodes not identified by T2 imaging (161 vs 114), improving detection of small nodal metastases. Therefore, DWI improves negative predictive value. Differentiation of benign and malignant subcentimeter nodes, however, is not possible with DWI.

Low accuracy for staging nodal metastases by conventional MR imaging has led to the study of novel detection techniques. Among these is the use of nanoparticle contrast media, such as ultrasmall superparamagnetic iron oxide (USPIO) particles. The magnetic properties of UPSIO particles generate changes in T2 and T2* signal intensity.

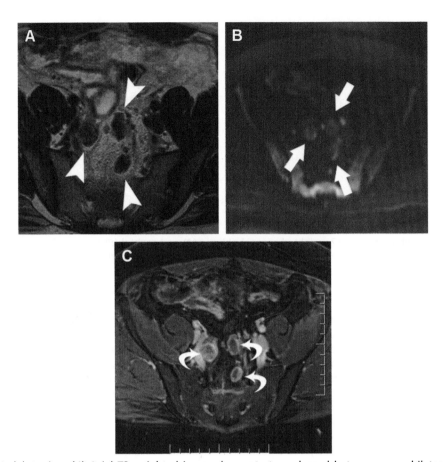

Fig. 18. Nodal staging. (*A*) Axial T2-weighted image demonstrates enlarged heterogeneous bilateral internal iliac lymph nodes (*arrowheads*). (*B*) High b-value (800) DWI shows restricted diffusion in each of the nodes (*arrows*). (*C*) Pathologic nodes also enhance heterogeneously on the dynamic contrast-enhanced sequence (*curved arrows*). The primary tumor (not shown) is inferior to the pathologic nodes.

In healthy lymph nodes, the particles are phagocytosed, leading to decreased T2 signal. Tumor cells prevent the uptake of nanoparticles, resulting in increased signal in involved nodes,[63] as in **Fig. 19.** More specific criteria have been proposed by Lahaye and colleagues,[64] suggesting that the most accurate and practical predictive criterion for malignancy is the percentage of white region in the node, with greater than 30% white region highly predictive of metastasis. More recently, a study by Koh and colleagues[65] concluded that use of USPIO particles improves specificity for malignant nodes but has the same sensitivity as morphologic characteristics on MR imaging. Use of USPIO particles is limited by availability in some countries and by timing considerations, because it must be administered 24 to 36 hours before performing the MR examination.

Gadofosveset is a gadolinium-based intravascular contrast agent that reversibly binds to albumin providing extended intravascular enhancement compared with existing extracellular MR contrast agents and was originally marketed as an MR angiography agent. More recently, studies by Lambregts and colleagues[66,67] have determined that imaging with Gadofosveset provides a high performance in diagnosis of malignant nodes. Benign nodes take up contrast, whereas malignant nodes do not. The uptake of contrast affects chemical shift artifact surrounding the nodes, with benign nodes demonstrating a characteristic nodal relief pattern. Although larger validation studies have not been completed, use of gadofosveset as a node-specific contrast agent may further increase the specificity of nodal staging by MR imaging (**Table 4**).

SPECIAL CONSIDERATIONS
Low Rectal Lesions

Low rectal cancers comprise approximately one-third of rectal cancers[68] and are generally defined as lowest margin of tumor less than 5 cm above the anal verge. Because of variability in length of

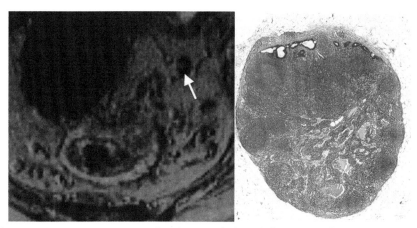

Fig. 19. (*Left*) Post-USPIOT2* MEDIC image showing a pathologic left mesorectal node, which shows a focus of eccentric nodal hyperintensity (*arrow*). Normal nodes are expected to show uniform signal darkening. (*Right*) The corresponding hematoxylin-eosin stain tissue of the pathologically matched lymph node shows subcapsular infiltration by adenocarcinoma. (*Courtesy of* Dr Dow-Mu Koh, MD, MRCP, FRCR, Sutton, Surrey, United Kingdom.)

the anal sphincter complex, there is inconsistent involvement of the anal sphincter complex in low rectal lesions. Relationship of tumor to anal sphincter complex and the ability of achieve clear distal margins not only determines the surgical approach but is key to success of surgery, because it is critical in achieving and good functional and oncologic outcome.

The anatomy of the low rectum differs from the mid- and upper-rectum in that the mesorectum tapers inferiorly toward the sphincter complex, resulting in a narrowing of the natural barrier to circumferential metastatic spread. MR imaging classification of low rectal tumors includes 2 categories, defined with respect to the relationship with the top border of the puborectalis muscle. Tumors in which the lowest extent of the tumor is above the top border of the puborectalis (levator insertion) are generally amenable to sphincter-sparing surgery. Tumors in which the inferior extent is at or below the top border of the puborectalis require either APR (T1 or early T2), extralevator APR (advanced T2 or T3), or pelvic exenteration (T4). For these tumors, the depth of invasion at or

Table 4
Rectal MR imaging report checklist: summary of important parameters meriting comment in the staging rectal MR imaging report

	Rectal MR Imaging Report Checklist	
Tumor	Size and location	Low, middle, high
	Appearance	Mucinous (yes or no)
	Circumferential extent	About clock face
	Distance from anal verge	In cm
	Distance from puborectalis (top of anal sphincter)	In cm
	Relationship to anterior peritoneal reflection	Above, at, below
	T category	T1–T4[a]
	EMVI	Absent, equivocal, present
CRM	Extramural depth of tumor invasion	Shortest distance
	Shortest distance from tumor to MRF	N/A if above peritoneal reflection
	Shortest distance from EMVI to MRF	In mm
	Shortest distance from satellite nodule to MRF	In mm
Node	Suspicious mesorectal lymph nodes	Size, heterogeneity, nonhomogeneous enhancement, USPIO characteristics
	Closest distance of suspicious node to MRF	In mm
	Location of lymph node closest to MRF	Above, at, or below tumor; about clock face
	Suspicious extramsorectal lymph nodes	Location

[a] MR findings for T stage summarized in **Table 3**.

below the puborectalis requires evaluation, with special attention to the involvement of the sphincter complex. If there is no definite involvement of the internal sphincter, T1 tumor is suspected. If the tumor is confined to the internal sphincter without involvement of intersphincteric fat, early T2 is suspected. If there is involvement of intersphincteric fat with possible or definite involvement of the external sphincter, late-stage T2 is suggested. If the lesion extends through the external sphincter without organ involvement, T3 is suggested, and if there is potential organ involvement, such as prostate or vagina, the tumor is a T4 lesion.

For tumors extending into the sphincter complex, survival and local recurrence rates after intersphincteric resection are similar to APR, and this procedure has replaced APR in selected patients.[69] Patients may qualify for intersphincteric APR (ie, ultra-LAR) if the intersphincteric plane is tumor-free and tumor does not extend within 1 mm of the outer border of the internal sphincter. If tumor extends into levator muscles, intersphincteric plane, and/or external sphincter, APR is generally required. Extensive local invasion requires single or multicompartmental pelvic exenteration. Surgical approaches are outlined in **Fig. 20** (**Table 5**).

Table 5 Special considerations for low rectal lesions	
T1	Tumor confined to submucosa, no involvement of internal sphincter
Early T2	Tumor confined to internal sphincter; no involvement of interspincteric fat
Advanced T2	Tumor involving intersphincteric fat, possible or definite involvement of external sphincter complex
T3	Tumor extending beyond external sphincter into surrounding soft tissue, no organ invasion
T3/possible T4	Possible involvement of adjacent organs (eg, prostate, vagina)
T4	Definite involvement of adjacent organs

Adapted from Al-Sukhni E, Milot L, Fruitman M, et al. User's Guide for the Synoptic MRI Report for Rectal Cancer. In: MacDonald B, Jhaveri J, Gill D, editors. Cancer Care Ontario. Retrieved from https://www.cancercare.on.ca/toolbox/SoPTools/sop_qi_resources/colorectal/.

Because the surgical approach is variable for the degree of sphincter complex involvement, it is incumbent on the radiologist to provide information on surgical planes available for resection. The depth of invasion for tumors at or below puborectalis should be described (**Figs. 21** and **22**). Examination of the sagittal and coronal images is essential to avoid the overstaging from apparent levator involvement on the axial images.[6] Several studies have shown that low rectal cancers requiring APR have worse outcome than those treated with LAR, considering margin involvement and perforation rates.[70–73] Margin positivity rates may be as high as 31.9%, despite neoadjuvant therapy in some cases.[74]

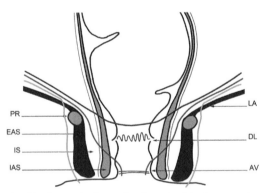

Fig. 20. Coronal schematic of anal sphincter complex depicting surgical dissection planes. Standard LAR (*blue*) leaves the pelvic floor muscles intact, and is the surgery of choice for mid- and high-rectal masses. APR (*green*) results in removal of the entire sphincter complex. Although standard APR typically tapers at the level of the pelvic floor resulting in a waist of the surgical plane, a more cylindrical approach that incorporates the levator musculature results in lower CRM positivity. Intersphincteric resection (*red*) sacrifices some or all of the internal anal sphincter, with the standard dissection plane at about the level of the dentate line. AV, anal verge; DL, dentate line; EAS, external sphincter complex; IAS, internal anal sphincter; IS, intersphincteric plane; LA, levator ani; PR, puborectalis.

Mucinous Lesions

Mucinous rectal carcinoma is a pathologic subtype of rectal adenocarcinoma characterized by production of extracellular mucin. These tumors tend to have a higher pathologic stage at the time of diagnosis, a greater tendency for metastasis, and local recurrence and unfavorable prognosis.[75] Identification of mucinous tumors is possible due to their intrinsic increased T2 signal relative to nonmucinous cancer. This may facilitate surgical management, because mucinous tumors are highly infiltrative (**Fig. 23**).

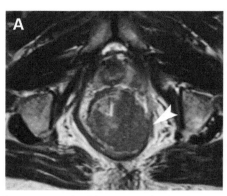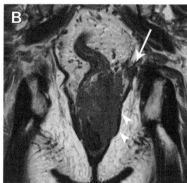

Fig. 21. Invasion to external sphincter complex in a low rectal lesion. Axial (*A*) and coronal (*B*) T2 images of a low rectal mass demonstrate contact of the left levator musculature (*arrowheads* [*B*]) and invasion through the external sphincter (*arrowhead* [*A*]). An involved mesorectal lymph node contacts the CRM (*arrow* [*B*]).

TREATMENT RESPONSE EVALUATION

The goal of neoadjuvant CCRT is downsizing and downstaging locally advanced tumor, with the intention of increasing the probability of complete resection, potentially allowing for sphincter preservation, and improving overall survival. The goal of imaging after neoadjuvant therapy depends on the strategy of the referring surgeon but generally includes evaluation for tumors most suitable for local excision, that is, identification of CRM involvement and tumors confined to the rectal wall.

The overall accuracy of MR imaging in restaging irradiated rectal cancers is much lower than initial staging MR imaging, with accuracies or 50% for T stage, 65% for N stage, and 66% for CRM.[76] High-resolution T2 images should be obtained. As of yet, no studies have shown improved accuracy with dynamic gadolinium-enhanced sequences.[77] Correlation with pretreatment images is essential, and ideally the images should be acquired in the same plane.[78] Comparison with initial staging MR images allows for assessment in changes of tumor bulk, location, and signal intensity. In addition to the characteristics assessed on the initial staging examination, several parameters should be discussed, including morphologic appearance of the tumor, length of tumor, and distance from anal verge. Depth of maximum extramural spread of tumor and fibrosis should be discussed separately. It is also of particular importance to comment on involvement of suspicious extramesorectal lymph nodes and possible anterior peritoneal reflection involvement at the time of restaging.[78]

Post–CCRT MR assessment may be imprecise from the point of view of overstaging, with understaging less common. Overstaging is caused by mural fibrosis and desmoplastic reaction caused or worsened by CCRT, manifested as hypointensity deep to the tumor that is imperceptible from it. There is also a tendency to overstage nodal metastases. Understaging is generally caused by residual nests of tumor cells within areas of T2 hypointense radiation fibrosis.[79] In general, understaging is less problematic, because surgery is completed with curative intent. An important corollary is the rare instance where surgical approach may be altered based on CR to treatment.[80–82] Evaluation of postneoadjuvant CCRT MR imaging for predicting CRM involvement has been studied by Vliegen and colleagues[83] and shown to have a high sensitivity (100%) but only moderate accuracy due to low specificity (32%–59%). The main limitation in post-therapy MR assessment is the differentiation of fibrotic tissue containing small nests of tumor cells from fibrotic tissue without

Fig. 22. Involvement of puborectalis. Axial T2 image of a low rectal lesion showing obliteration of the intersphincteric plane and invasion of the puborectalis posteriorly (*arrow*). Internal anal sphincter (*arrowhead*). P, puborectalis; V, vagina.

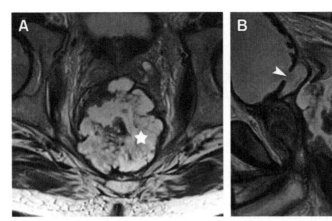

Fig. 23. Axial (*A*) and coronal (*B*) T2-weighted images of a large mucinous tumor. Note the areas of marked T2 hyperintensity within the lesion (*star [A, B]*), indicative of mucin pools. Incidental bladder diverticulum (*arrowhead [B]*).

residual malignant cells. The study investigators concluded that fibrotic areas should be considered potentially invaded, resulting in overstaging and low PPV, because overstaging of disease is much more acceptable and because understaging may lead to incomplete tumor resection and an unacceptably high risk of local tumor.

MR imaging assessment of both tumor morphology and volume post-CCRT is an accurate predictor of residual tumor limited to bowel wall. Volumetric assessment of tumors pre- and postneoadjuvant treatment can help predict tumor confined to rectal wall at the time of surgery. In a small study by Dresen and colleagues,[84] all tumors greater than 50 cm^3 with greater than 75% reduction in volume post-CCRT were confined to the rectal wall. This result helps reduce overstaging due to peritumoral fibrosis in postneoadjuvant therapy patients on conventional MR sequences, which may further tailor patient therapy. Although this could allow clinicians to consider transanal local excision in good responders after radiation therapy with concomitant chemotherapy, with less morbidity and mortality than after standard surgery, this approach is controversial.

Dynamic contrast-enhanced MR imaging has been evaluated in the restaging of rectal cancer. Pretreatment perfusion index values and slope of contrast medium enhancement curve help identify responders. Accuracy and reproducibility, however, have not been established, and this is not currently recommended for routine restaging.[78] Dynamic contrast enhancement has been shown, however, to increase accuracy for the assessment of nodal disease at the time of restaging. T2 hypointensity of lymph nodes and early complete arterial enhancement are predictive findings of benign nodes, whereas T2 heterogeneity and incomplete arterial enhancement are indicators of malignant nodal disease.[85]

DWI in Post-CCRT Patients

Because morphologic evaluation of complete response (CR) is difficult due to poor differentiation of small residual tumor from radiation fibrosis, concurrent evaluation of high b-value DWIs using pre- and post-treatment ADC values improves overall performance of diagnosing CR after neoadjuvant therapy.[86] Tumor should remain hyperintense on DWI, and the presence of hyperintensity within the treated lesion suggests residual disease. Because fibrosis typically has low cellular density, it demonstrates low signal on high b-value diffusion imaging. Similarly, because apoptosis progresses in tumor cells during CCRT, diffusion restriction decreases accordingly. The higher cellular density and unorganized cellular structure of residual tumor results in increased signal on high b-value sequences. In 2009, a single-center study by Kim and colleagues[87] showed DWI in addition to standard MR imaging showed significant performance improvement in diagnosing CR, a finding substantiated in a more recent multicenter trial by Lambregts and colleagues.[88] In these studies, there was decreased tendency for overstaging of simple fibrosis. Interpretation errors in the study by Lambregts and colleagues remained, however, problematic, resulting in a sensitivity of only 52% to 64%. For this reason, DWI is more useful in excluding CR than predicting it. Furthermore, the prediction of CR by imaging is most useful in institutions where referring surgeons may opt for minimally invasive surgery or a wait-and-see approach for complete responders.

Qualitative evaluation of post-treatment ADC performed by several groups has also shown that low-baseline ADC values and reduction in ADC after treatment correspond with good pathologic response to CRT.[89–91] As an adjunct, several groups have assessed change in ADC values during neoadjuvant treatment. A small study performed by Kremser and colleagues[92] determined that patients with a good treatment response showed increased ADC values in the first week of treatment, with subsequent sustained decrease. Nonresponders did not have a similar ADC increase in the early stage of treatment. A subsequent study by Sun and colleagues[93] was

in agreement, but another study by Engin and colleagues[94] found no difference in ADC values between partial and complete responders.

DWI has also been used to predict response to treatment and tumor aggressiveness. At initial staging MR imaging, a high ADC value corresponds to rapid diffusion in the necrotic area of a cancer and indicates a more aggressive tumor. This predicts a poor response to CCRT.[93,95,96]

Examination of quantitative ADC values has shown mixed results. Use of quantitative ADC is not advisable as routine, because current software algorithms for ADC value calculation preclude reproducible measurements across vendor

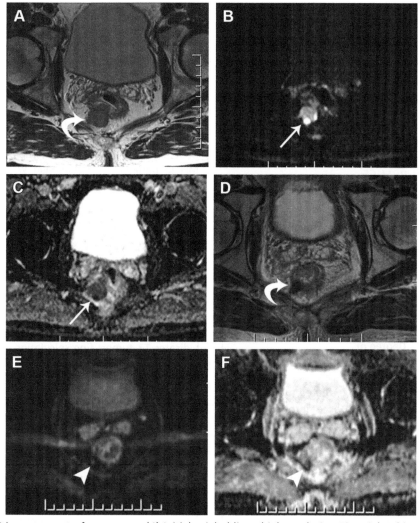

Fig. 24. DWI in assessment of recurrence. (*A*) Initial axial oblique high-resolution T2-weighted image shows an advanced T3 stage with large nodular extramural component (*curved arrow*). (*B*) High b-value DWI (b = 800) demonstrates hyperintensity in this component of the tumor (*arrow* [*B*]) and (*C*) hypointensity on ADC map (*arrow* [*C*]). (*D*) Post-treatment axial oblique T2 weighted image. The tumor is replaced by hypointense fibrotic tissue (*curved arrow* [*D*]), and it is difficult to determine if there is a small amount of viable tumor within fibrosis. (*E*) Post-treatment DWI image with (*F*) ADC map reveals a tiny residual focus of hyperintensity (*arrowhead* [*E*]), with larger area of low ADC signal (*arrowhead* [*F*]).

platforms. The utility of DWI in the setting of prediction or evaluation of tumor response is as yet undetermined due to the paucity of published research, requiring interpretive caution outside academic setting, particularly when patient management is altered (**Fig. 24**).[97]

Mucinous adenocarcinoma generally has a poor response to neoadjuvant therapy. It also remains T2 hyperintense after treatment, rendering post-CCRT MR assessment particularly difficult.[98]

Treatment response cannot be assessed with DWI in mucinous tumors, due to inherent hyperintensity of ADC in these tumors pretreatment.[28] Mucin may also be identified within initially nonmucinous tumors at the time of restaging MR imaging as a consequence of treatment.

It has also been shown that patients with more fibrosis on surgical specimen post–neoadjuvant therapy have improved survival relative to patients with less fibrosis[99] and that tumor regression grade is an independent predictor of overall and disease-free survival.[78] The MR imaging classification of tumor regression grade is outlined in **Table 6**; although MR imaging and pathologic classification are similar, they are not the same.

LOCAL RECURRENCE

More than half of pelvic recurrences occur in the first 2 years after resection, with the vast majority detected by 4 years. Risk factors for local recurrence include tumor stage, grade, distance from anal verge, lymphovascular invasion, CRM positivity, surgical technique, anastomotic leak, and perforation at the time of surgery. Patients with recurrence may be candidates for surgery with curative intent or palliative radiation and/or surgery. Although CT is routinely used for imaging surveillance, CT cannot reliably differentiate between postsurgical and postradiation change from recurrent disease, relying more often on changes in size and morphology of soft tissue masses in the pelvis over time.[100] MR also has limitations in this regard, particularly in the postoperative period. Although T2 hyperintensity is often seen in recurrent tumor, the finding is not specific and can be seen in non-neoplastic inflammation or edema, sometimes persisting for up to 2 years after surgery. High T2 signal has a low specificity and cannot aid the differentiation of recurrence from benign scar.[101] Mature fibrosis generally demonstrates decreased T2 signal but may harbor microscopic foci of tumor, and apparent fibrosis cannot exclude recurrent disease.[102] Hence, evaluation of T2 images alone is insufficient for the detection of recurrence due to low specificity.[103] Differentiation of recurrent rectal cancer from postsurgical and postradiotherapy changes on MR is particularly problematic when assessing the pelvic sidewalls.[104] Dynamic contrast-enhanced MR imaging is a useful technique in the evaluation of local recurrence. Several groups

Table 6
Radiologic MR imaging classification of tumor regression grade

Tumor Regression Grade	Degree of Response	Description
1	Complete	No evidence of ever treated tumor
2	Good	Dense fibrosis/mucin; no obvious residual tumor
3	Moderate	>50% Fibrosis/mucin and visible intermediate signal
4	Slight	Little areas of fibrosis/mucin; mostly tumor
5	None	Same appearance and signal as original tumor

Data from Taylor FG, Swift RI, Blomqvist L, et al. A systematic approach to the interpretation of preoperative staging MRI for rectal cancer. AJR Am J Roentgenol 2008;191(6): 1827–35.

Box 1
Pearls and pitfalls

Ulcerating tumors causing erosion of muscularis propria may result in extramural depth of invasion discordance between MR and histology.

A broad-based bulge beyond muscular layer indicates T3 tumor; fine spiculation beyond the muscular wall may be due to peritumoral fibrosis or tumor infiltration.

Angulation of the axial plane orthogonal to the tumor is critical for staging in order to have distinct margins of the outer muscular layer.

Examination of the sagittal and coronal images is essential for low rectal tumors to avoid overstaging from apparent levator involvement on the axial images and to provide information regarding available surgical dissection planes.

Use of DWI plays a role in the assessment of treatment response in post-CCRT patients but is more useful in excluding disease response than predicting it.

Dynamic contrast-enhanced MR imaging is a useful technique in the evaluation of local recurrence.

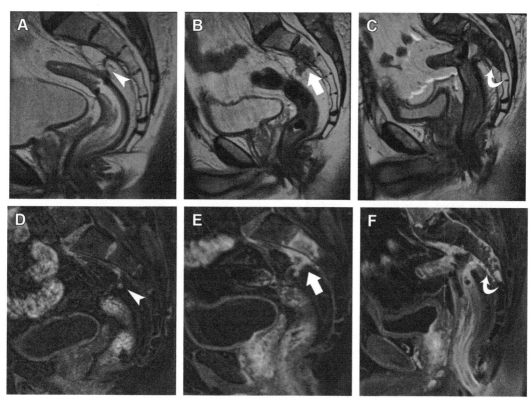

Fig. 25. Local anastomotic recurrence. Sagittal T2-weighted images (*A–C*) and T1 gradient-echo gadolinium-enhanced images (*D–F*) demonstrate progression of local recurrence over 10 months. Initially, a tiny area of T2 hypointense fibrosis is noted, with minimal corresponding enhancement, which could represent postoperative granulation tissue (*arrowheads [A, D]*). (*B, E*) Six months later, there is a larger area of low-intermediate T2 signal, infiltrating the S2 segment (*arrow [B]*) with rim enhancement suggestive of recurrence (*arrow [E]*). Ten months after the initial study, more extensive marrow signal abnormality and peripheral enhancement is evident (*curved arrows [C, F]*). Involvement of the S1 segment excludes the possibility of pelvic exenteration.

Table 7
What the referring clinician needs to know

Surgical oncologist	What is the relationship of tumor to CRM?	Threatened surgical margin necessitates neoadjuvant therapy.
	What is the relationship of tumor to the sphincter complex?	Involvement of sphincter alters surgical approach and gives information on available planes for dissection, allowing for attempts at sphincter preservation and continuity of colon.
	What is the location of suspicious lymph nodes?	Surgical objective is complete tumor and nodal excision.
Radiation oncologist	What is the location of suspicious extramesorectal lymph nodes?	Conformal techniques for RT require mapping of nodal metastases beyond intended radiation field in mesorectum.
Medical oncologist	Is there evidence of distant metastatic disease?	Metastatic disease at presentation may require alteration in approach to treatment.
All	Does tumor extend beyond muscularis propria? Are poor prognostic features present (extramural depth of invasion <5 mm, EMVI)?	No significant survival benefit for T1, T2, and favorable early T3 lesions, with potential morbidity from neoadjuvant CCRT.

have demonstrated that recurrent tumor enhances earlier than benign postoperative and postradiation change, due to increased regional blood flow and vascular permeability.[103,105,106] Additionally, a heterogeneous pattern of enhancement is more suggestive of recurrent disease than of benign changes. Rim enhancement may be seen but is less specific in the recent postoperative period, because pelvic abscess may have a similar appearance. MR imaging has been shown to be highly accurate in assessing disease extent in cases of known recurrence,[107] an important factor in identifying cases that are potentially resectable with curative intent. Indications for curative surgery are specific and include involvement of S1/S2 nerve roots, sacral invasion above S2/S3, encasement of iliac vessels, and extension through the greater sciatic notch (**Box 1, Fig. 25, Table 7**).[108,109]

SUMMARY

In the age of multidisciplinary approach to rectal cancer treatment, radiologists play an important and expanding role as members of a multidisciplinary team. Preventing over- and undertreatment requires a preoperative prediction of risk for local recurrence tailor neoadjuvant therapy for each patient, which is accomplished with staging MR imaging. In addition to TNM staging, MR imaging provides additional prognostic information by assessment of extramural depth of invasion, EVMI, and CRM, affirming its essential role in the preoperative assessment of rectal cancer. As conservative management techniques (ie, wait-and-see approach) become more clinically relevant, MR imaging with DWI will continue to play an expanding role in the assessment of treatment response.

REFERENCES

1. Maier A, Fuchsjager M. Preoperative staging of rectal cancer. Eur J Radiol 2003;47(2):89–97.
2. Siegel R, Naishadham D, Jemal A. Cancer statistics, 2013. CA Cancer J Clin 2013;63(1):11–30.
3. Sauer R, Becker H, Hohenberger W, et al. Preoperative versus postoperative chemoradiotherapy for rectal cancer. N Engl J Med 2004;351(17): 1731–40.
4. Heald RJ, Moran BJ, Ryall RD, et al. Rectal cancer: the Basingstoke experience of total mesorectal excision, 1978-1997. Arch Surg 1998;133(8): 894–9.
5. Enker WE. Total mesorectal excision–the new golden standard of surgery for rectal cancer. Ann Med 1997;29(2):127–33.
6. Shihab OC, Moran BJ, Heald RJ, et al. MRI staging of low rectal cancer. Eur Radiol 2009;19(3):643–50.
7. Kosinski L, Habr-Gama A, Ludwig K, et al. Shifting concepts in rectal cancer management: a review of contemporary primary rectal cancer treatment strategies. CA Cancer J Clin 2012;62(3):173–202.
8. Hermanek P, Junginger T. The circumferential resection margin in rectal carcinoma surgery. Tech Coloproctol 2005;9(3):193–9 [discussion: 199–200].
9. Quirke P, Durdey P, Dixon MF, et al. Local recurrence of rectal adenocarcinoma due to inadequate surgical resection. Histopathological study of lateral tumour spread and surgical excision. Lancet 1986;2(8514):996–9.
10. Garcia-Aguilar J, Pollack J, Lee SH, et al. Accuracy of endorectal ultrasonography in preoperative staging of rectal tumors. Dis Colon Rectum 2002; 45(1):10–5.
11. Fernandez-Esparrach G, Ayuso-Colella JR, Sendino O, et al. EUS and magnetic resonance imaging in the staging of rectal cancer: a prospective and comparative study. Gastrointest Endosc 2011; 74(2):347–54.
12. Cartana ET, Parvu D, Saftoiu A. Endoscopic ultrasound: current role and future perspectives in managing rectal cancer patients. J Gastrointestin Liver Dis 2011;20(4):407–13.
13. Beets-Tan RG, Beets GL. Rectal cancer: review with emphasis on MR imaging. Radiology 2004; 232(2):335–46.
14. Bipat S, Glas AS, Slors FJ, et al. Rectal cancer: local staging and assessment of lymph node involvement with endoluminal US, CT, and MR imaging–a meta-analysis. Radiology 2004;232(3): 773–83.
15. Maizlin ZV, Brown JA, So G, et al. Can CT replace MRI in preoperative assessment of the circumferential resection margin in rectal cancer? Dis Colon Rectum 2010;53(3):308–14.
16. Brown G, Richards CJ, Newcombe RG, et al. Rectal carcinoma: thin-section MR imaging for staging in 28 patients. Radiology 1999;211(1): 215–22.
17. Brown G, Daniels IR, Richardson C, et al. Techniques and trouble-shooting in high spatial resolution thin slice MRI for rectal cancer. Br J Radiol 2005;78(927):245–51.
18. Kaur H, Choi H, You YN, et al. MR imaging for preoperative evaluation of primary rectal cancer: practical considerations. Radiographics 2012;32(2): 389–409.
19. Kim H, Lim JS, Choi JY, et al. Rectal cancer: comparison of accuracy of local-regional staging with two- and three-dimensional preoperative 3-T MR imaging. Radiology 2010;254(2):485–92.
20. Hori M, Kim T, Onishi H, et al. Uterine tumors: comparison of 3D versus 2D T2-weighted turbo spin-echo

MR imaging at 3.0 T–initial experience. Radiology 2011;258(1):154–63.

21. Blomqvist L, Holm T, Rubio C, et al. Rectal tumours–MR imaging with endorectal and/or phased-array coils, and histopathological staging on giant sections. A comparative study. Acta Radiol 1997; 38(3):437–44.

22. Dewhurst C, Rosen MP, Blake MA, et al. ACR Appropriateness Criteria pretreatment staging of colorectal cancer. J Am Coll Radiol 2012;9(11): 775–81.

23. Brown G, Daniels IR. Preoperative staging of rectal cancer: the MERCURY research project. Recent Results Cancer Res 2005;165:58–74.

24. Suzuki C, Torkzad MR, Tanaka S, et al. The importance of rectal cancer MRI protocols on interpretation accuracy. World J Surg Oncol 2008;6:89.

25. MERCURY Study Group. Extramural depth of tumor invasion at thin-section MR in patients with rectal cancer: results of the MERCURY study. Radiology 2007;243(1):132–9.

26. Rao SX, Zeng MS, Chen CZ, et al. The value of diffusion-weighted imaging in combination with T2-weighted imaging for rectal cancer detection. Eur J Radiol 2008;65(2):299–303.

27. Ichikawa T, Erturk SM, Motosugi U, et al. High-B-value diffusion-weighted MRI in colorectal cancer. AJR Am J Roentgenol 2006;187(1):181–4.

28. Lim KS, Tan CH. Diffusion-weighted MRI of adult male pelvic cancers. Clin Radiol 2012;67(9): 899–908.

29. Mizukami Y, Ueda S, Mizumoto A, et al. Diffusion-weighted magnetic resonance imaging for detecting lymph node metastasis of rectal cancer. World J Surg 2011;35(4):895–9.

30. Jao SY, Yang BY, Weng HH, et al. Evaluation of gadolinium-enhanced T1-weighted magnetic resonance imaging in the preoperative assessment of local staging in rectal cancer. Colorectal Dis 2010;12(11):1139–48.

31. Vliegen RF, Beets GL, von Meyenfeldt MF, et al. Rectal cancer: MR imaging in local staging–is gadolinium-based contrast material helpful? Radiology 2005;234(1):179–88.

32. Brown G, Kirkham A, Williams GT, et al. High-resolution MRI of the anatomy important in total mesorectal excision of the rectum. AJR Am J Roentgenol 2004; 182(2):431–9.

33. Dujovny N, Quiros RM, Saclarides TJ. Anorectal anatomy and embryology. Surg Oncol Clin N Am 2004;13(2):277–93.

34. Gollub MJ, Maas M, Weiser M, et al. Recognition of the anterior peritoneal reflection at rectal MRI. AJR Am J Roentgenol 2013;200(1):97–101.

35. Salerno G, Daniels IR, Moran BJ, et al. Clarifying margins in the multidisciplinary management of

rectal cancer: the MERCURY experience. Clin Radiol 2006;61(11):916–23.

36. Klessen C, Rogalla P, Taupitz M. Local staging of rectal cancer: the current role of MRI. Eur Radiol 2007;17(2):379–89.

37. Zhang XM, Zhang HL, Yu D, et al. 3-T MRI of rectal carcinoma: preoperative diagnosis, staging, and planning of sphincter-sparing surgery. AJR Am J Roentgenol 2008;190(5):1271–8.

38. Beets-Tan RG, Beets GL, Borstlap AC, et al. Preoperative assessment of local tumor extent in advanced rectal cancer: CT or high-resolution MRI? Abdom Imaging 2000;25(5):533–41.

39. Taylor FG, Swift RI, Blomqvist L, et al. A systematic approach to the interpretation of preoperative staging MRI for rectal cancer. AJR Am J Roentgenol 2008;191(6):1827–35.

40. Brown G, Radcliffe AG, Newcombe RG, et al. Preoperative assessment of prognostic factors in rectal cancer using high-resolution magnetic resonance imaging. Br J Surg 2003;90(3): 355–64.

41. Compton CC, Greene FL. The staging of colorectal cancer: 2004 and beyond. CA Cancer J Clin 2004; 54(6):295–308.

42. Beets-Tan RG, Beets GL, Vliegen RF, et al. Accuracy of magnetic resonance imaging in prediction of tumour-free resection margin in rectal cancer surgery. Lancet 2001;357(9255):497–504.

43. Willett CG, Badizadegan K, Ancukiewicz M, et al. Prognostic factors in stage T3N0 rectal cancer: do all patients require postoperative pelvic irradiation and chemotherapy? Dis Colon Rectum 1999; 42(2):167–73.

44. Cawthorn SJ, Parums DV, Gibbs NM, et al. Extent of mesorectal spread and involvement of lateral resection margin as prognostic factors after surgery for rectal cancer. Lancet 1990;335(8697): 1055–9.

45. Merkel S, Mansmann U, Siassi M, et al. The prognostic inhomogeneity in pT3 rectal carcinomas. Int J Colorectal Dis 2001;16(5):298–304.

46. Pollheimer MJ, Kornprat P, Pollheimer VS, et al. Clinical significance of pT sub-classification in surgical pathology of colorectal cancer. Int J Colorectal Dis 2010;25(2):187–96.

47. Taylor FG, Quirke P, Heald RJ, et al. Preoperative high-resolution magnetic resonance imaging can identify good prognosis stage I, II, and III rectal cancer best managed by surgery alone: a prospective, multicenter, European study. Ann Surg 2011;253(4):711–9.

48. Beaumont C, Pandey T, Gaines Fricke R, et al. MR evaluation of rectal cancer: current concepts. Curr Probl Diagn Radiol 2013;42(3):99–112.

49. Taylor FG, Quirke P, Heald RJ, et al. One millimetre is the safe cut-off for magnetic resonance imaging

prediction of surgical margin status in rectal cancer. Br J Surg 2011;98(6):872–9.

50. Horn A, Dahl O, Morild I. Venous and neural invasion as predictors of recurrence in rectal adenocarcinoma. Dis Colon Rectum 1991;34(9):798–804.

51. Smith NJ, Barbachano Y, Norman AR, et al. Prognostic significance of magnetic resonance imaging-detected extramural vascular invasion in rectal cancer. Br J Surg 2008;95(2):229–36.

52. Engelen SM, Beets-Tan RG, Lahaye MJ, et al. Location of involved mesorectal and extramesorectal lymph nodes in patients with primary rectal cancer: preoperative assessment with MR imaging. Eur J Surg Oncol 2008;34(7):776–81.

53. Wang C, Zhou ZG, Yu YY, et al. Patterns of lateral pelvic lymph node metastases and micrometastases for patients with lower rectal cancer. Eur J Surg Oncol 2007;33(4):463–7.

54. Luna-Perez P, Corral P, Labastida S, et al. Inguinal lymph node metastases from rectal adenocarcinoma. J Surg Oncol 1999;70(3):177–80.

55. Sugihara K, Kobayashi H, Kato T, et al. Indication and benefit of pelvic sidewall dissection for rectal cancer. Dis Colon Rectum 2006;49(11):1663–72.

56. Dworak O. Number and size of lymph nodes and node metastases in rectal carcinomas. Surg Endosc 1989;3(2):96–9.

57. Kotanagi H, Fukuoka T, Shibata Y, et al. The size of regional lymph nodes does not correlate with the presence or absence of metastasis in lymph nodes in rectal cancer. J Surg Oncol 1993;54(4):252–4.

58. Brown G, Richards CJ, Bourne MW, et al. Morphologic predictors of lymph node status in rectal cancer with use of high-spatial-resolution MR imaging with histopathologic comparison. Radiology 2003;227(2):371–7.

59. Kim JH, Beets GL, Kim MJ, et al. High-resolution MR imaging for nodal staging in rectal cancer: are there any criteria in addition to the size? Eur J Radiol 2004;52(1):78–83.

60. Matsuoka H, Nakamura A, Sugiyama M, et al. MRI diagnosis of mesorectal lymph node metastasis in patients with rectal carcinoma. What is the optimal criterion? Anticancer Res 2004;24(6):4097–101.

61. Koh DM, Brown G, Temple L, et al. Distribution of mesorectal lymph nodes in rectal cancer: in vivo MR imaging compared with histopathological examination. Initial observations. Eur Radiol 2005;15(8):1650–7.

62. Mir N, Sohaib SA, Collins D, et al. Fusion of high b-value diffusion-weighted and T2-weighted MR images improves identification of lymph nodes in the pelvis. J Med Imaging Radiat Oncol 2010;54(4):358–64.

63. Will O, Purkayastha S, Chan C, et al. Diagnostic precision of nanoparticle-enhanced MRI for lymph-node metastases: a meta-analysis. Lancet Oncol 2006;7(1):52–60.

64. Lahaye MJ, Beets GL, Engelen SM, et al. Locally advanced rectal cancer: MR imaging for restaging after neoadjuvant radiation therapy with concomitant chemotherapy. Part II. What are the criteria to predict involved lymph nodes? Radiology 2009;252(1):81–91.

65. Koh DM, George C, Temple L, et al. Diagnostic accuracy of nodal enhancement pattern of rectal cancer at MRI enhanced with ultrasmall superparamagnetic iron oxide: findings in pathologically matched mesorectal lymph nodes. AJR Am J Roentgenol 2010;194(6):W505–13.

66. Lambregts DM, Beets GL, Maas M, et al. Accuracy of gadofosveset-enhanced MRI for nodal staging and restaging in rectal cancer. Ann Surg 2011;253(3):539–45.

67. Lambregts DM, Heijnen LA, Maas M, et al. Gadofosveset-enhanced MRI for the assessment of rectal cancer lymph nodes: predictive criteria. Abdom Imaging 2013;38(4):720–7.

68. Salerno G, Daniels IR, Brown G, et al. Variations in pelvic dimensions do not predict the risk of circumferential resection margin (CRM) involvement in rectal cancer. World J Surg 2007;31(6):1313–20.

69. Akagi Y, Shirouzu K, Ogata Y, et al. Oncologic outcomes of intersphincteric resection without preoperative chemoradiotherapy for very low rectal cancer. Surg Oncol 2013;22(2):144–9.

70. Kapiteijn E, Marijnen CA, Nagtegaal ID, et al. Preoperative radiotherapy combined with total mesorectal excision for resectable rectal cancer. N Engl J Med 2001;345(9):638–46.

71. Nagtegaal ID, van de Velde CJ, Marijnen CA, et al. Low rectal cancer: a call for a change of approach in abdominoperineal resection. J Clin Oncol 2005;23(36):9257–64.

72. Guillou PJ, Quirke P, Thorpe H, et al. Short-term endpoints of conventional versus laparoscopic-assisted surgery in patients with colorectal cancer (MRC CLASICC trial): multicentre, randomised controlled trial. Lancet 2005;365(9472):1718–26.

73. Marr R, Birbeck K, Garvican J, et al. The modern abdominoperineal excision: the next challenge after total mesorectal excision. Ann Surg 2005;242(1):74–82.

74. Shihab OC, Brown G, Daniels IR, et al. Patients with low rectal cancer treated by abdominoperineal excision have worse tumors and higher involved margin rates compared with patients treated by anterior resection. Dis Colon Rectum 2010;53(1):53–6.

75. Hussain SM, Outwater EK, Siegelman ES. Mucinous versus nonmucinous rectal carcinomas: differentiation with MR imaging. Radiology 1999;213(1):79–85.

76. Kim DJ, Kim JH, Lim JS, et al. Restaging of rectal cancer with mr imaging after concurrent chemotherapy and radiation therapy. Radiographics 2010;30(2):503–16.

77. Kim SH, Lee JM, Park HS, et al. Accuracy of MRI for predicting the circumferential resection margin, mesorectal fascia invasion, and tumor response to neoadjuvant chemoradiotherapy for locally advanced rectal cancer. J Magn Reson Imaging 2009;29(5):1093–101.

78. Patel UB, Blomqvist LK, Taylor F, et al. MRI after treatment of locally advanced rectal cancer: how to report tumor response–the MERCURY experience. AJR Am J Roentgenol 2012;199(4): W486–95.

79. Del Vescovo R, Trodella LE, Sansoni I, et al. MR imaging of rectal cancer before and after chemoradiation therapy. Radiol Med 2012;117(7):1125–38.

80. Kuo LJ, Chern MC, Tsou MH, et al. Interpretation of magnetic resonance imaging for locally advanced rectal carcinoma after preoperative chemoradiation therapy. Dis Colon Rectum 2005;48(1):23–8.

81. Chen CC, Lee RC, Lin JK, et al. How accurate is magnetic resonance imaging in restaging rectal cancer in patients receiving preoperative combined chemoradiotherapy? Dis Colon Rectum 2005;48(4):722–8.

82. Valentini V, Coco C, Cellini N, et al. Preoperative chemoradiation for extraperitoneal T3 rectal cancer: acute toxicity, tumor response, and sphincter preservation. Int J Radiat Oncol Biol Phys 1998; 40(5):1067–75.

83. Vliegen RF, Beets GL, Lammering G, et al. Mesorectal fascia invasion after neoadjuvant chemotherapy and radiation therapy for locally advanced rectal cancer: accuracy of MR imaging for prediction. Radiology 2008;246(2):454–62.

84. Dresen RC, Beets GL, Rutten HJ, et al. Locally advanced rectal cancer: MR imaging for restaging after neoadjuvant radiation therapy with concomitant chemotherapy. Part I. Are we able to predict tumor confined to the rectal wall? Radiology 2009;252(1):71–80.

85. Alberda WJ, Dassen HP, Dwarkasing RS, et al. Prediction of tumor stage and lymph node involvement with dynamic contrast-enhanced MRI after chemoradiotherapy for locally advanced rectal cancer. Int J Colorectal Dis 2013;28(4):573–80.

86. Lambrecht M, Vandecaveye V, De Keyzer F, et al. Value of diffusion-weighted magnetic resonance imaging for prediction and early assessment of response to neoadjuvant radiochemotherapy in rectal cancer: preliminary results. Int J Radiat Oncol Biol Phys 2012;82(2): 863–70.

87. Kim SH, Lee JM, Hong SH, et al. Locally advanced rectal cancer: added value of diffusion-weighted MR imaging in the evaluation of tumor response to neoadjuvant chemo- and radiation therapy. Radiology 2009;253(1):116–25.

88. Lambregts DM, Vandecaveye V, Barbaro B, et al. Diffusion-weighted MRI for selection of complete responders after chemoradiation for locally advanced rectal cancer: a multicenter study. Ann Surg Oncol 2011;18(8):2224–31.

89. Hein PA, Kremser C, Judmaier W, et al. Diffusion-weighted magnetic resonance imaging for monitoring diffusion changes in rectal carcinoma during combined, preoperative chemoradiation: preliminary results of a prospective study. Eur J Radiol 2003;45(3):214–22.

90. Intven M, Reerink O, Philippens ME. Diffusion-weighted MRI in locally advanced rectal cancer: pathological response prediction after neoadjuvant radiochemotherapy. Strahlenther Onkol 2013;189(2):117–22.

91. Jung SH, Heo SH, Kim JW, et al. Predicting response to neoadjuvant chemoradiation therapy in locally advanced rectal cancer: diffusion-weighted 3 Tesla MR imaging. J Magn Reson Imaging 2012;35(1):110–6.

92. Kremser C, Judmaier W, Hein P, et al. Preliminary results on the influence of chemoradiation on apparent diffusion coefficients of primary rectal carcinoma measured by magnetic resonance imaging. Strahlenther Onkol 2003;179(9):641–9.

93. Sun YS, Zhang XP, Tang L, et al. Locally advanced rectal carcinoma treated with preoperative chemotherapy and radiation therapy: preliminary analysis of diffusion-weighted MR imaging for early detection of tumor histopathologic downstaging. Radiology 2010;254(1):170–8.

94. Engin G, Sharifov R, Gural Z, et al. Can diffusion-weighted MRI determine complete responders after neoadjuvant chemoradiation for locally advanced rectal cancer? Diagn Interv Radiol 2012;18(6):574–81.

95. DeVries AF, Kremser C, Hein PA, et al. Tumor microcirculation and diffusion predict therapy outcome for primary rectal carcinoma. Int J Radiat Oncol Biol Phys 2003;56(4):958–65.

96. Dzik-Jurasz A, Domenig C, George M, et al. Diffusion MRI for prediction of response of rectal cancer to chemoradiation. Lancet 2002;360(9329): 307–8.

97. Boone D, Taylor SA, Halligan S. Diffusion weighted MRI: overview and implications for rectal cancer management. Colorectal Dis 2013; 15(6):655–61.

98. Grillo-Ruggieri F, Mantello G, Berardi R, et al. Mucinous rectal adenocarcinoma can be associated to tumor downstaging after preoperative chemoradiotherapy. Dis Colon Rectum 2007;50(10): 1594–603.

99. Dworak O, Keilholz L, Hoffmann A. Pathological features of rectal cancer after preoperative radiochemotherapy. Int J Colorectal Dis 1997;12(1): 19–23.

100. Thompson WM, Halvorsen RA, Foster WL Jr, et al. Preoperative and postoperative CT staging of rectosigmoid carcinoma. AJR Am J Roentgenol 1986;146(4):703–10.

101. Ebner F, Kressel HY, Mintz MC, et al. Tumor recurrence versus fibrosis in the female pelvis: differentiation with MR imaging at 1.5 T. Radiology 1988; 166(2):333–40.

102. Glazer HS, Lee JK, Levitt RG, et al. Radiation fibrosis: differentiation from recurrent tumor by MR imaging. Radiology 1985;156(3):721–6.

103. Kinkel K, Tardivon AA, Soyer P, et al. Dynamic contrast-enhanced subtraction versus T2-weighted spin-echo MR imaging in the follow-up of colorectal neoplasm: a prospective study of 41 patients. Radiology 1996;200(2):453–8.

104. Messiou C, Chalmers AG, Boyle K, et al. Pre-operative MR assessment of recurrent rectal cancer. Br J Radiol 2008;81(966):468–73.

105. Muller-Schimpfle M, Brix G, Layer G, et al. Recurrent rectal cancer: diagnosis with dynamic MR imaging. Radiology 1993;189(3):881–9.

106. Dicle O, Obuz F, Cakmakci H. Differentiation of recurrent rectal cancer and scarring with dynamic MR imaging. Br J Radiol 1999;72(864):1155–9.

107. Robinson P, Carrington BM, Swindell R, et al. Recurrent or residual pelvic bowel cancer: accuracy of MRI local extent before salvage surgery. Clin Radiol 2002;57(6):514–22.

108. Messiou C, Chalmers A, Boyle K, et al. Surgery for recurrent rectal carcinoma: the role of preoperative magnetic resonance imaging. Clin Radiol 2006; 61(3):250–8.

109. Sagar PM, Pemberton JH. Surgical management of locally recurrent rectal cancer. Br J Surg 1996; 83(3):293–304.

Magnetic Resonance Imaging of Penile Cancer

Sumit Gupta, PhD, MRCP[a,b,]*, Arumugam Rajesh, MBBS, FRCR[a]

KEYWORDS

- Penile cancer • MR imaging • Penile imaging • Staging

KEY POINTS

- Penile cancer, although rare in the developed world, has devastating physical and psychological consequences for the patient.
- MR imaging accurately delineates the penile anatomy and is the imaging modality of choice of accurate local staging of primary penile cancer.
- Novel MR imaging techniques such as lymphotropic nanoparticle-enhanced MR imaging may help identify metastatic lymph node disease.

INTRODUCTION

Penile cancer is a rare neoplasm with devastating physical and psychological consequences for patients. There is a wide regional variation in the incidence of penile cancer throughout the world ranging from less than 1 case per 100,000 men in Europe and the United States, to 8.3 cases per 100,000 in Brazil, to even higher in Uganda.[1] In the United States, it is estimated that there will be 1640 new cases of penile cancer and 320 cancer-related deaths in 2014.[2] Penile cancer tends to be a disease of older men. There is an abrupt increase in incidence in men aged approximately 60 years and the incidence peaks in men aged 80 years.

This article reviews the normal penile anatomy, MR imaging techniques for evaluation of the penis, and MR imaging features of primary and metastatic penile cancer. Recent advances in penile cancer imaging are discussed.

ANATOMY

The anatomy of the penis has important implications for the diagnosis and treatment of penile cancer. The penis can be divided into root and body. The root of the penis is located in the superficial perineal pouch and is the primary fixation point. The body of the penis is composed of three tubular endothelium-lined cavernous structures: paired corpora cavernosa, located on the dorsolateral aspect of the penis, and a single corpora spongiosum located in the midline ventrally (**Fig. 1**). The corpus spongiosum contains the urethra and extends anteriorly to form the glans penis. The three corpora of the penis are covered by three connective tissue layers. The innermost layer is fibrous tunica albuginea. The middle layer is the Buck fascia, a fibrous layer that surrounds the corpora cavernosa and separates them from corpora spongiosum. External to this is a layer of loose connective tissue that is covered by dartos fascia.

Disclosure: This review article presents independent research funded by the National Institute for Health Research (NIHR). The views expressed are those of the authors and not necessarily those of the NHS, the NIHR, or the Department of Health (S. Gupta).
[a] Department of Radiology, University Hospitals of Leicester NHS Trust, Leicester General Hospital, Gwendolen Road, Leicester LE5 4PW, UK; [b] University of Leicester, Glenfield Hospital, Groby Road, Leicester LE3 9QP, UK
* Corresponding author. University of Leicester, Glenfield Hospital, Groby Road, Leicester LE3 9QP, UK.
E-mail address: drsumitgupta@yahoo.com

Magn Reson Imaging Clin N Am 22 (2014) 191–199
http://dx.doi.org/10.1016/j.mric.2014.01.005
1064-9689/14/$ – see front matter © 2014 Elsevier Inc. All rights reserved.

mri.theclinics.com

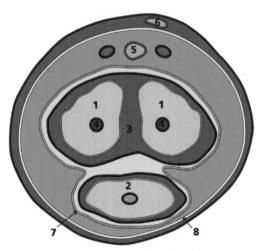

Fig. 1. Normal penile anatomy (*axial view*). 1, corpora cavernosa; 2, corpus spongiosum; 3, tunica albuginea; 4, cavernosal arteries; 5, deep dorsal vein; 6, superficial dorsal vein; 7, Buck fascia; 8, dartos fascia.

MR IMAGING

Patient positioning is paramount in MR imaging of the penis. Patient is imaged in a supine position. To elevate the scrotum and penis, a folded towel is placed between the patient's legs. The penis is taped to the abdomen in a dorsiflexed position to prevent movement and pulsation artifacts. A surface coil is placed on the penis to improve signal-to-noise ratio.

Scardino and colleagues[3] suggested that MR imaging with artificial erection, achieved by injecting 10 μg of prostaglandin E1 into the corpus cavernosum, provides a more robust local staging of the penile cancer. Artificial erection is routinely used at the authors' institute for MR imaging of the penis. However, this is avoided if there is large and painful penile tumor because of the increased risk of priapism. The MR imaging sequences used are (1) T1-axial images of the pelvis, which provide an overview of the pelvis and lymph nodes and (2) T2-axial, sagittal, and coronal images of the penis (**Box 1**). Gadolinium-enhanced sequences are not routinely used at the authors' institute. The three corpora of the penis demonstrate intermediate T1 and high T2 signal on MR imaging. Relative to the corpus spongiosum, the muscular wall of the urethra appears hypointense on both T1-weighted and T2-weighted sequences. Tunica albuginea, Buck fascia, and dartos fascia show low signal intensity on all MR imaging sequences. Tunica albuginea and Buck fascia cannot reliably be differentiated on MR imaging and appear as a hypointense rim of tissue around the corpora. T2-weighted imaging demonstrates a greater

degree of contrast between the corpora and tunica albuginea. MR imaging appearances of normal penis are summarized in **Table 1** and illustrated in **Fig. 2**.

MR IMAGING OF PENILE CANCER
Primary Tumor Imaging

Most penile cancers are squamous cell carcinomas (SCCs). Other reported histologic types of penile malignancies consist of basal cell carcinoma, melanoma, sarcoma, and metastatic lesions. Moreover, several histologic subtypes of SCC have been described, each with unique clinicopathologic characteristics and outcome features.[4,5] The most common histologic subtype of penile carcinoma is the usual-type SCC.[6] Most penile tumors originate from the mucosal surface extending from the preputial orifice to the meatus urethralis.[6] Tumors arising from the glans penis

---

Box 1
MR imaging protocol for penile cancer

Adequate patient positioning.

Artificial erection: injection of 10 μg of prostaglandin E1 into the corpus cavernosum.

MR imaging Acquisition Parameters[a]	TR	TE	FOV
T1 Axial Pelvis	679	12	400[b]
T2 Axial Penis	5720	97	350
T2 Sagittal Penis	3750	100	250
T2 Coronal Penis	3750	100	250

Abbreviations: FOV, field of view; TE, echo time; TR, repetition time.
   [a] MR imaging acquisition parameters at the authors' institute.
   [b] Variable based on patient body habitus.

Table 1
MR appearance of the normal penis

	T1-Weighted MR Imaging	T2-Weighted MR Imaging
Dartos fascia	Hypointense	Hypointense
Tunica albuginea and Buck fascia	Hypointense	Hypointense
Muscular wall of the urethra	Hypointense[a]	Hypointense[a]
Corpora cavernosa and corpus spongiosum	Intermediate	High signal

[a] Hypointense relative to corpus spongiosum.

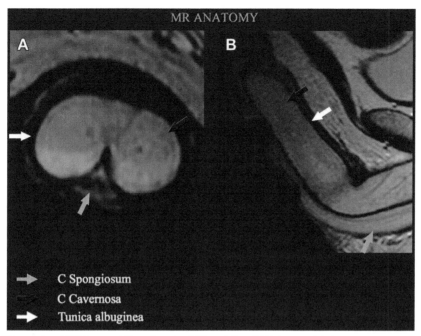

Fig. 2. Axial T2-weighted MR image (A) and sagittal T2-weighted MR image (B) show corpora cavernosa, corpus spongiosum, and tunica albuginea.

are more common than are those involving the foreskin or the sulcus.[6,7] A recent study of about 5000 cases of invasive penile carcinoma showed that the primary site of disease was the glans penis in 34.5% of cases, prepuce in 13.2%, shaft in 5.3%, and overlapping in 4.5%, with primary site unspecified in 42.5% of cases.[8] MR imaging is the most sensitive imaging modality for local staging of penile cancer because of its exceptional soft-tissue resolution, multiplanar capability, and excellent spatial resolution in the assessment of superficial structures. On MR imaging, primary penile cancers usually appear as solitary, ill-defined, and infiltrating mass lesions that are hypointense relative to the adjacent corpora on both T1-weighted and T2-weighted images.[9] MR imaging enables accurate assessment of the local extent of the penile lesion, depth of tumor invasion, and involvement of tunica albuginea and other adjacent structures, including corpora, urethra, or scrotal skin. The international tumor node metastasis (TNM) staging system for penile cancer was last updated in 2009[10] and is used for staging the primary tumor (Fig. 3, Table 2). MR imaging and histology appearances of various T stages of penile cancer are illustrated in Figs. 4–7.

Penile metastatic lesions are rare and most frequently occur from primary tumors in the genitourinary tract or the recto-sigmoid region.

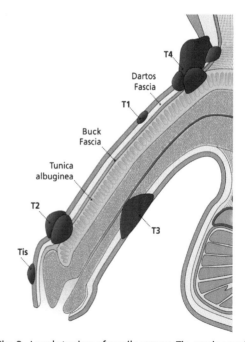

Fig. 3. Local staging of penile cancer. Tis, carcinoma in situ; T1, tumor invades subepithelial connective tissue; T2, tumor invades corpus spongiosum or corpora cavernosa; T3, tumor invades urethra; T4, tumor invades other adjacent structures.

Table 2
TNM classification of penile cancer (2009)

T—Primary Tumor		
TX		Primary tumor cannot be assessed
T0		No evidence of primary tumor
Tis		Carcinoma in situ
Ta		Noninvasive verrucous carcinoma, not associated with destructive invasion
T1	T1a	Tumor invades subepithelial connective tissue without lymph vascular invasion and is not poorly differentiated
	T1b	Tumor invades subepithelial connective tissue with lymph vascular invasion or is poorly differentiated
T2		Tumor invades corpus spongiosum or corpora cavernosa
T3		Tumor invades urethra
T4		Tumor invades other adjacent structures
N—Regional Lymph Nodes (Clinical)[a]		
cNX		Regional lymph nodes cannot be assessed
cN0		No palpable or visibly enlarged inguinal lymph nodes
cN1		Palpable mobile unilateral inguinal lymph nodes
cN2		Palpable mobile multiple or bilateral inguinal lymph nodes
cN3		Fixed inguinal nodal mass or pelvic lymphadenopathy, unilateral or bilateral
N—Regional Lymph Nodes (Pathologic)[b]		
pNX		Regional lymph nodes cannot be assessed
pN0		No regional lymph metastasis
pN1		Metastasis in a single inguinal lymph node
pN2		Metastasis in multiple or bilateral inguinal lymph nodes
pN3		Extranodal extension of lymph node metastasis or pelvic lymph nodes, unilateral or bilateral
M—Distant Metastasis		
M0		No distant metastasis
M1		Distant metastasis (includes lymph node metastasis outside the true pelvis)

[a] Clinical stage definition based on palpation and imaging.
[b] Pathologic stage definition based on biopsy of surgical excision.
From Edge S, Byrd DR, Compton CC, et al. AJCC cancer staging manual. New York: Springer; 2010.

However, penile metastases from stomach, lung, and thyroid cancers have been described.[11,12] The most common lesions to metastasize to the penis are prostate and bladder cancers.[9,13] Penile metastatic lesions can be difficult to differentiate from primary penile lesions on MR imaging. Typically, they are seen as multiple masses in the corpora cavernosa and corpus spongiosum where lesions demonstrate low signal intensity compared with to normal corporal tissue on both T1-weighted and T2-weighted images (see **Fig. 6**B).[13]

Lymph Node Imaging

The most important prognostic factor for survival in patients with penile cancer is the presence and extent of inguinal lymph node involvement.[14] Determining the extent of lymph node involvement influences treatment strategy.[15] Based on the location of the primary tumor, the site of lymph node metastasis can be predicted. Skin and prepuce lymphatics drain into the superficial inguinal lymph nodes, the glans drains into the deep inguinal and external iliac nodes, and corpora and penile urethra drains into the internal iliac nodes. Clinical examination and conventional imaging methods, including ultrasound, CT, and MR imaging, are unreliable in detecting lymph node metastasis. At the time of initial diagnosis up to 30% to 60% of patients with SCC have palpable inguinal lymph nodes,[16] approximately half of which are reactive.[17] Sensitivity of clinical staging of the lymph nodes have been shown to be 40% to 60% with a false-negative rate between 10% and 20%.[18,19] Abnormal lymph nodes on CT and MR imaging are determined based of lymph node size, which results in underdetection of occult metastasis in normal-sized lymph nodes and increase in false-positive rates in patients with enlarged lymph nodes secondary to infection or inflammation. However, cross-section imaging can detect enlarged retroperitoneal and pelvic lymph nodes not identified by clinical examination.

Prophylactic lymphadenopathy has been shown to improve long-term survival.[19–21] Recently, Ornellas and colleagues[14] have shown a disease-free survival rate of 71% for subjects who underwent immediate lymphadenectomy compared with those who had a delayed lymphadenectomy with a disease-free survival rate of 30%. However, universal use of this procedure would result in overtreatment in 60% to 75% of patients.[22] Moreover, it has been reported that inguinal lymphadenectomy is associated with major morbidity, including lymphedema, skin flap necrosis, and a 1% to 3% mortality rate.[22–25] However, refinement of surgical techniques has reduced the

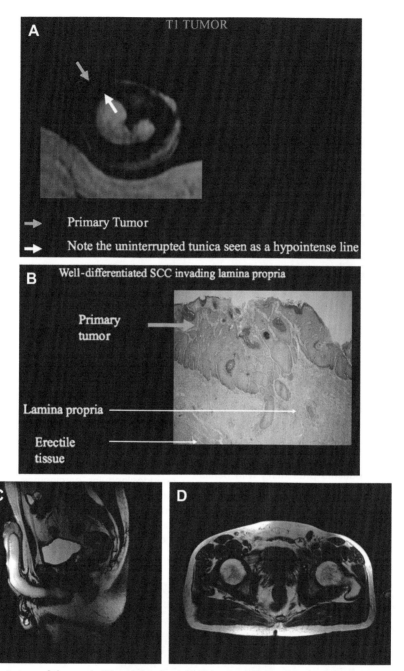

Fig. 4. T1 primary tumor of the penis. T2-weighted axial MR image (*A*) showing the primary tumor and an uninterrupted tunica albuginea. Histologic specimen (*B*) from the same patient showing well-differentiated SCC invading the lamina propria. Another patient with sagittal T2-weighted MR image of the penis (*C*) and axial T1-weighted MR image of the pelvis (*D*) showing small irregular mass involving the glans penis with intact tunica albuginea and an enlarged left inguinal lymph node (radiological classification: T1, N1).

complication rate by 50%.[15,26] Reduction in postoperative morbidity has also been achieved by using video endoscopic inguinal lymphadenectomy.[27] Novel techniques such as dynamic sentinel lymph node biopsy result in 70% reduction in the need for radical lymph node dissection,[28,29] which remains the current gold standard for diagnosis of lymph node metastasis.

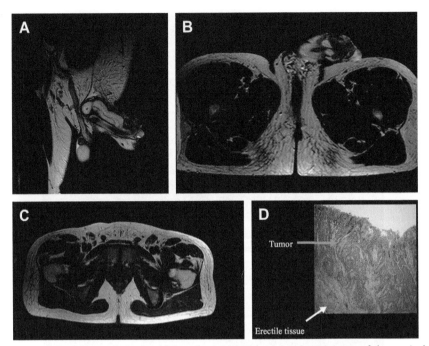

Fig. 5. T2 primary tumor of the penis. Sagittal (*A*) and axial (*B*) T2-weighted MR images of the penis showing mass originating from the glans penis. This mass is disrupting the tunica albuginea and invading the corpora cavernosa on both sides. Axial T1-weighted MR image of the pelvis (*C*) demonstrates bilateral enlarged inguinal lymph nodes (radiological classification: T2, N2). Histologic specimen (*D*) from the same patient showing moderately differentiated SCC with invasion into corpora cavernosa.

Distant Metastasis Imaging

Less than 3% of patients presenting with penile cancer have metastasis.[30] The lungs, liver, and retroperitoneum are the most common sites of metastasis. Distant metastasis generally occurs late in the course of the disease and is associated with a poor prognosis. The histologic subtypes of penile SCC that are aggressive with high metastatic rates are basaloid, sarcomatoid, and pseudoglandular carcinomas.[6] Adenosquamous carcinomas frequently metastasize to the inguinal lymph nodes but have a good prognosis. CT is the modality of choice for evaluation of distant metastases.

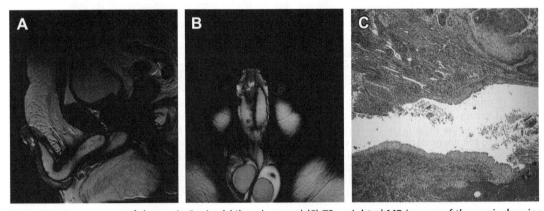

Fig. 6. T3 primary tumor of the penis. Sagittal (*A*) and coronal (*B*) T2-weighted MR images of the penis showing soft tissue mass arising in the region of the glans penis and involving the corpus spongiosum and urethra. There is a 6 mm nodule in the right corpora cavernosa. No enlarged inguinal or pelvic lymph nodes were seen (radiological classification: T3, N0, M1). Histologic specimen (*C*) from the same patient showing invasion of the urethra by the penile SCC.

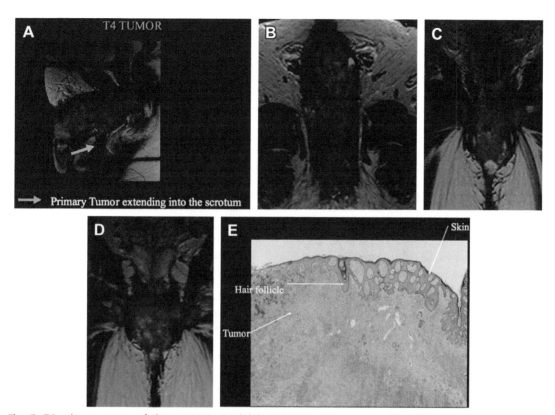

Fig. 7. T4 primary tumor of the penis. Sagittal (*A*) and coronal (*B–D*) T2-weighted MR images of the penis showing penile tumor extending into the scrotum (*A*) and prostate gland (*C, D*). Histologic specimen (*E*) from the same patient showing sarcomatoid SCC invading testicular skin.

Novel MR Imaging Techniques

Lymphotropic nanoparticle-enhanced MR imaging has emerged as a promising technique for regional lymph node staging of penile[31] and various other cancers.[32–35] This technique uses an infusion of coated ultrasmall iron oxide particles, which are taken up homogeneously by functioning macrophages in normal lymph nodes and demonstrate low signal on gradient echo T2*-weighted images, with only the center being spared in lymph nodes with hilar fat. Metastatic lymph nodes lack the normal phagocytes needed to take up the nanoparticles[36] and hence have high signal intensity on gradient echo T2*-weighted images. Using this technique, Tabatabaei and colleagues[31] demonstrated a sensitivity and specificity of 100% and 97%, respectively, for detection of inguinal lymph node involvement in subjects with penile cancer after assessment of 113 lymph nodes in seven subjects.

SUMMARY

MR imaging is the modality of choice for accurate local staging of penile cancer. Moreover, penile MR imaging helps detect lymph node involvement and metastatic disease of the penis. Familiarity with optimal imaging protocols, normal penile anatomy, and MR imaging appearances is essential for the radiologist. Emerging techniques may further enhance the abilities of MR imaging to detect lymph node metastasis.

REFERENCES

1. Pizzocaro G, Algaba F, Horenblas S, et al. EAU penile cancer guidelines 2009. Eur Urol 2010;57: 1002–12.
2. Siegel R, Ma J, Zou Z, et al. Cancer statistics, 2014. CA Cancer J Clin 2014;64:9–29.
3. Scardino E, Villa G, Bonomo G, et al. Magnetic resonance imaging combined with artificial erection for local staging of penile cancer. Urology 2004;63: 1158–62.
4. Cubilla AL, Reuter V, Velazquez E, et al. Histologic classification of penile carcinoma and its relation to outcome in 61 patients with primary resection. Int J Surg Pathol 2001;9:111–20.
5. Guimaraes GC, Cunha IW, Soares FA, et al. Penile squamous cell carcinoma clinicopathological

features, nodal metastasis and outcome in 333 cases. J Urol 2009;182:528–34 [discussion: 34].

6. Chaux A, Velazquez EF, Algaba F, et al. Developments in the pathology of penile squamous cell carcinomas. Urology 2010;76:S7–14.

7. Pow-Sang MR, Benavente V, Pow-Sang JE, et al. Cancer of the penis. Cancer Control 2002;9: 305–14.

8. Hernandez BY, Barnholtz-Sloan J, German RR, et al. Burden of invasive squamous cell carcinoma of the penis in the United States, 1998–2003. Cancer 2008;113:2883–91.

9. Vossough A, Pretorius ES, Siegelman ES, et al. Magnetic resonance imaging of the penis. Abdom Imaging 2002;27:640–59.

10. Edge SB, Byrd DR, Compton CC, et al. AJCC cancer staging manual. 7th edition. New York: Springer; 2010.

11. Grimm MO, Spiegelhalder P, Heep H, et al. Penile metastasis secondary to follicular thyroid carcinoma. Scand J Urol Nephrol 2004;38:253–5.

12. Perdomo JA, Hizuta A, Iwagaki H, et al. Penile metastasis secondary to cecum carcinoma: a case report. Hepatogastroenterology 1998;45:1589–92.

13. Demuren OA, Koriech O. Isolated penile metastasis from bladder carcinoma. Eur Radiol 1999;9: 1596–8.

14. Ornellas AA, Kinchin EW, Nobrega BL, et al. Surgical treatment of invasive squamous cell carcinoma of the penis: Brazilian National Cancer Institute long-term experience. J Surg Oncol 2008;97: 487–95.

15. Bevan-Thomas R, Slaton JW, Pettaway CA. Contemporary morbidity from lymphadenectomy for penile squamous cell carcinoma: the M.D. Anderson Cancer Center Experience. J Urol 2002; 167:1638–42.

16. Horenblas S. Lymphadenectomy for squamous cell carcinoma of the penis. Part 1: diagnosis of lymph node metastasis. BJU Int 2001;88:467–72.

17. Abi-Aad AS, deKernion JB. Controversies in ilioinguinal lymphadenectomy for cancer of the penis. Urol Clin North Am 1992;19:319–24.

18. Catalona WJ. Modified inguinal lymphadenectomy for carcinoma of the penis with preservation of saphenous veins: technique and preliminary results. J Urol 1988;140:306–10.

19. McDougal WS. Carcinoma of the penis: improved survival by early regional lymphadenectomy based on the histological grade and depth of invasion of the primary lesion. J Urol 1995;154:1364–6.

20. McDougal WS. Advances in the treatment of carcinoma of the penis. Urology 2005;66:114–7.

21. Theodorescu D, Russo P, Zhang ZF, et al. Outcomes of initial surveillance of invasive squamous cell carcinoma of the penis and negative nodes. J Urol 1996;155:1626–31.

22. Solsona E, Iborra I, Rubio J, et al. Prospective validation of the association of local tumor stage and grade as a predictive factor for occult lymph node micrometastasis in patients with penile carcinoma and clinically negative inguinal lymph nodes. J Urol 2001;165:1506–9.

23. Ornellas AA, Seixas AL, Marota A, et al. Surgical treatment of invasive squamous cell carcinoma of the penis: retrospective analysis of 350 cases. J Urol 1994;151:1244–9.

24. Johnson DE, Lo RK. Management of regional lymph nodes in penile carcinoma. Five-year results following therapeutic groin dissections. Urology 1984;24:308–11.

25. Ornellas AA, Seixas AL, de Moraes JR. Analyses of 200 lymphadenectomies in patients with penile carcinoma. J Urol 1991;146:330–2.

26. Nelson BA, Cookson MS, Smith JA Jr, et al. Complications of inguinal and pelvic lymphadenectomy for squamous cell carcinoma of the penis: a contemporary series. J Urol 2004;172:494–7.

27. Tobias-Machado M, Tavares A, Ornellas AA, et al. Video endoscopic inguinal lymphadenectomy: a new minimally invasive procedure for radical management of inguinal nodes in patients with penile squamous cell carcinoma. J Urol 2007;177:953–7 [discussion: 8].

28. Kroon BK, Horenblas S, Meinhardt W, et al. Dynamic sentinel node biopsy in penile carcinoma: evaluation of 10 years experience. Eur Urol 2005;47:601–6 [discussion: 6].

29. Hegarty PK, Kayes O, Freeman A, et al. A prospective study of 100 cases of penile cancer managed according to European Association of Urology guidelines. BJU Int 2006;98:526–31.

30. Rippentrop JM, Joslyn SA, Konety BR. Squamous cell carcinoma of the penis: evaluation of data from the surveillance, epidemiology, and end results program. Cancer 2004;101:1357–63.

31. Tabatabaei S, Harisinghani M, McDougal WS. Regional lymph node staging using lymphotropic nanoparticle enhanced magnetic resonance imaging with ferumoxtran-10 in patients with penile cancer. J Urol 2005;174:923–7 [discussion: 7].

32. Deserno WM, Harisinghani MG, Taupitz M, et al. Urinary bladder cancer: preoperative nodal staging with ferumoxtran-10-enhanced MR imaging. Radiology 2004;233:449–56.

33. Keller TM, Michel SC, Frohlich J, et al. USPIO-enhanced MRI for preoperative staging of gynecological pelvic tumors: preliminary results. Eur Radiol 2004;14:937–44.

34. Anzai Y, Piccoli CW, Outwater EK, et al. Evaluation of neck and body metastases to nodes with ferumoxtran 10-enhanced MR imaging: phase III safety and efficacy study. Radiology 2003;228: 777–88.

35. Harisinghani MG, Barentsz J, Hahn PF, et al. Nonin-
    vasive detection of clinically occult lymph-node me-
    tastases in prostate cancer. N Engl J Med 2003;348:
    2491–9.

36. Harisinghani MG, Dixon WT, Saksena MA, et al. MR
    lymphangiography: imaging strategies to optimize
    the imaging of lymph nodes with ferumoxtran-10.
    Radiographics 2004;24:867–78.

Magnetic Resonance Imaging of Pelvic Metastases in Male Patients

Seyed Mahdi Abtahi, MD, Yun Mao, MD,
Duangkamon Prapruttam, MD, Azadeh Elmi, MD,
Sandeep S. Hedgire, MD*

KEYWORDS

- Pelvic metastases • MR imaging • Nodal metastases • Skeletal metastases
- Peritoneal metastases

KEY POINTS

- Lymph node involvement signifies an adverse prognosis and modifies the treatment strategies. The number and regions of affected pelvic nodes directly influence the survival rate.
- Superior soft tissue resolution of magnetic resonance (MR) imaging aids in detection of metastatic lesions to visceral organs and detects nonpalpable lesions of the prostate, penis, and testes.
- Disseminated tumors commonly seed pelvic recesses lined by parietal peritoneum, followed by accumulation of increasing amounts of ascites in the bilateral paravesical recesses.
- MR imaging offers better characterization of musculoskeletal metastasis compared with computed tomography and conventional radiography.
- With diffusion-weighted imaging and nanoparticle-enhanced MR imaging there is an impending paradigm shift from structural to functional imaging.

INTRODUCTION

The pelvis is a common site for primary and metastatic tumors. Diagnosis of pelvic metastatic lesions is a crucial step in the staging of primary cancer because it implies an adverse prognosis. Magnetic resonance (MR) imaging is a noninvasive imaging tool for diagnosis of pelvic metastasis based on its multiplanar imaging capability and excellent soft tissue resolution. In addition, MR imaging can also differentiate between different tissue elements including characterization of vascular and nonvascular structures without contrast.[1] Knowledge of basic MR signal characteristics of normal (**Figs. 1–5, Table 1**) and abnormal structures is essential for accurate interpretation of pelvic MR imaging. This article provides a concise overview of nodal, visceral, and musculoskeletal metastatic lesions affecting the pelvis and their MR imaging characteristics.[2]

LYMPH NODE METASTASIS

In most patients with known pelvic malignancies, presence of nodal disease signifies adverse prognosis and dictates treatment strategies. The number and regions of the pelvic nodes involved affect the nodal (N) and metastasis (M) staging of the tumor and also influence the survival rate. Understanding the lymphatic drainage pathways and MR diagnostic criteria of abnormal nodes can help in the evaluation of pelvic lymph node metastasis.[3]

Pelvic Lymphatic Metastatic Pathways

The primary lymphatic drainage in the male pelvis includes 4 pathways: (1) the anterior route, draining lymph from the anterior wall of the bladder to the internal iliac (hypogastric) nodes; (2) the lateral

Division of Abdominal Imaging and Interventional Radiology, Massachusetts General Hospital, 55 Fruit Street, White 270, Boston, MA 02114, USA
* Corresponding author.
E-mail address: hedgire.sandeep@mgh.harvard.edu

Magn Reson Imaging Clin N Am 22 (2014) 201–215
http://dx.doi.org/10.1016/j.mric.2014.01.006
1064-9689/14/$ – see front matter © 2014 Elsevier Inc. All rights reserved.

mri.theclinics.com

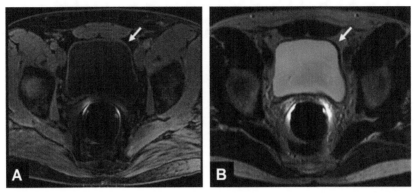

Fig. 1. Normal urinary bladder. (A) Axial T1-weighted image shows intermediate signal intensity of urinary bladder wall (*arrow*). (B) Axial T2-weighted image shows low signal intensity of urinary bladder wall (*arrow*).

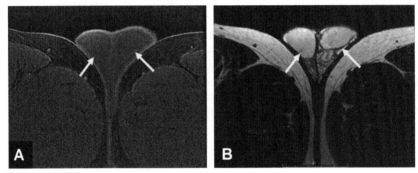

Fig. 2. Normal testicles. (A) Axial T1-weighted image shows homogeneous intermediate signal intensity of bilateral testicles (*arrows*). (B) Axial T2-weighted image shows high signal intensity of both testicles (*arrows*).

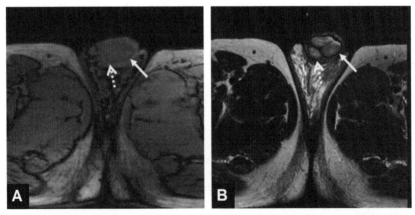

Fig. 3. Normal penis. (A) Axial T1-weighted image shows intermediate signal intensity of the corpus cavernosum (*arrow*) and spongiosum (*dotted arrow*). (B) Axial T2-weighted image shows high signal intensity of the corpus spongiosum (*dotted arrow*) and heterogeneous signal intensity of the corpus cavernosum (*arrow*).

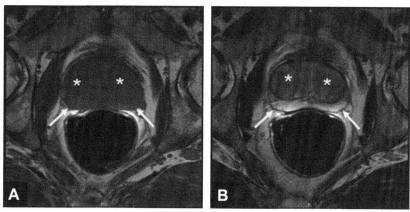

Fig. 4. Normal prostate gland. (*A*) Axial T1-weighted image shows low to intermediate signal intensity of the prostate gland. (*B*) Axial T2-weighted image provides distinction between the heterogeneous central gland (*asterisks*) and the high signal intensity of peripheral zones (*arrows*).

route, draining lymph from pelvic organs to the external iliac nodal group; (3) the internal iliac (hypogastric) route, draining lymph to the junctional nodes located at the junction between the internal and external iliac vessels; and (4) the presacral route, draining lymph to the common iliac nodes. To a great extent, the location of the primary tumor (bladder, prostate, testes, and penis) and integrity of the draining lymphatics determine which pathway is predominantly affected. The location of the involved lymph nodes can be attributed to N or M stage; for example, inguinal nodes are considered as regional metastasis for penile cancer but distant metastasis for prostate cancer. Familiarity with these lymphatic metastatic pathways is crucial for pelvic node evaluation.[4]

Prostate Cancer

The lymphatic drainage of prostate cancer involves the obturator, presacral, hypogastric, and external iliac nodes and further to the common iliac and para-aortic nodes. The main drainage pathway is the lateral route, which involves nodes located along the lateral aspect of the external iliac artery, and the sentinel nodes are the obturator nodes. From there, the tumor may further spread to the nodes located medial and posterior to the external iliac vein. The second most common pathway is the internal iliac route, via the nodes located along the visceral branches of the internal iliac vessels, and the corresponding sentinel nodes are located at the junction of the internal and external iliac vessels.[4,5] Following therapeutic irradiation of the prostate or radical prostatectomy, recurrent metastatic disease is most often seen in extrapelvic nodes. The survival rate depends on the number of positive nodes. The 10-year disease-free survival in cases of solitary nodal involvement is 70%, compared with 49% for multiple (more than 5) nodes.[6]

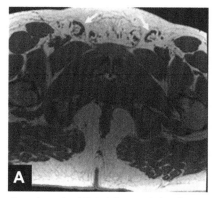
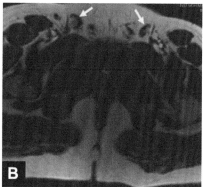

Fig. 5. Benign lymph node. (*A*) Axial T1-weighted image and (*B*) axial T2-weighted image show benign appearance of bilateral small inguinal lymph nodes (*arrow*) with preserved central fatty hila.

Table 1
Normal appearance of male pelvic organ on MR imaging

Organ	T1 Appearance	T2 Appearance
Bladder wall	Intermediate signal	Low signal intensity
Testicles	Homogeneous intermediate signal intensity	High signal intensity relative to skeletal muscle
Epididymis	Isointense to the testis	Lower signal intensity than the testis
Tunica albuginea	Low signal intensity	Low signal intensity
Corpora cavernosa and spongiosa	Intermediate signal intensity	Corpus spongiosum shows homogeneous high signal intensity Corpora cavernosa may have a heterogeneous signal intensity
Prostate	Low to intermediate signal intensity	Glandular tissue normally shows high signal intensity, whereas fibromuscular stromal elements have low signal intensity
Bone marrow	Hematopoietic marrow equal to or slightly higher than muscle	The same as T1
Muscle	Intermediate between fat and cortical bone	Intermediate between fat and cortical bone

Penile Cancer

The lymph node metastasis of penile cancer commonly involves the nodes in the superficial and deep inguinal regions, and subsequently the pelvic lymph nodes associated with ipsilateral iliac vessels and obturator fossa are also affected. The saphenofemoral junction node is the sentinel node for penile cancer.[4] Greater number of metastatic nodes, bilateral disease, and deep pelvic nodal metastases adversely affect prognosis. The mortality increases from 25% in cases of low-volume inguinal metastases to 75% in patients with more than 2 nodes. In patients with penile carcinoma, nodal metastases at the time of diagnosis can be seen in 22% to 61% of patients.[7]

Testicular Cancer

Testicular cancer spreads via the para-aortic pathway, with lymphatic drainage following the gonadal vessels to the retroperitoneum, whereas metastases in pelvic nodes are rare except in epididymal cancer. As the volume of the tumor increases, the metastasis may further spread from retroperitoneal nodes to the common iliac, internal iliac, and external iliac nodes.[4] More importantly, because of disruption of the normal lymphatic drainage pathways after orchiectomy, the pelvic and inguinal nodes should be assessed as regional nodes.[8,9] The spread of testicular cancer is most commonly by means of lymphatic metastasis. The evaluation of nodal status dictates the of

postorchidectomy radiation and helps in assessing treatment response. MR imaging is especially useful in this regard because patients with seminomas are often young adults and have a good 5-year survival rate (>80%).[4,5,10]

In testicular cancer, unlike many other malignancies, the lymph nodes should be measured by calculating the maximum diameter of the lymph node as opposed to the short-axis of the lymph node.[4,5]

Bladder Carcinoma

Bladder carcinoma commonly spreads via a pelvic pathway and the specific sites of primary tumors determine the pathway. For tumors located in the fundus of the bladder, the most common sites of metastasis are the obturator and internal iliac nodes; for upper and lower lateral wall tumors, the external iliac nodes are predominantly affected; and for bladder neck cancers, node metastasis spreads from the presacral nodes to the common iliac nodes.[4] However, radical cystectomy for bladder cancer can change the pathways and, in such circumstances, clinicians should carefully evaluate the common iliac and para-aortic nodes.[11] The metastatic lymph nodes below the level of the common iliac vessels are categorized as regional metastasis, whereas the nodes above the level of common iliac vessels are categorized as distant metastasis.[5] Similar to penile neoplasm, as the number of nodes involved increases, the survival rate of bladder cancer decreases. Three-year survival in node-negative patients is approximately 70%; in patients with solitary positive node it is approximately 50%, and it is reduced to approximately 25% if multiple nodes are involved.[12,13]

Rectal Cancer

Rectal lymph drainage follows 3 pathways depending on the sites of primary tumors: (1) upper rectum, to the inferior mesenteric nodes followed by the para-aortic nodes; (2) middle rectum, to the obturator and hypogastric nodes; (3) lower rectum, to the inguinal nodes.[14]

In T3 rectal tumors, survival in lymph node–negative patients is approximately 70%, compared with 35% in lymph node–positive patients, and survival in patients with 1 to 3 nodes involved is significantly better than in those with more than 3 nodes.[15,16]

Metastatic pelvic side wall (PSW) nodes on MR imaging represent a more advanced disease state in rectal cancer (Fig. 5). The obturator fossa is the predominant site for PSW node metastasis. Among patients undergoing primary surgery, PSW node involvement suspected on MR imaging is associated with worse 5-year disease-free survival compared with no suspected PSW node involvement: 31% versus 76%.[17]

Diagnostic Criteria

Multiplanar MR imaging has shown an accuracy of 90%, a positive predictive value of 94%, and a negative predictive value of 89% in the detection of nodal metastasis in bladder and prostate cancer.[18] For conventional MR imaging, the morphologic criteria, including size, shape, contour, fatty hilum, signal abnormalities, and location, are currently followed in clinical practice (Table 2).

Nodal size

Nodal size is the main criteria to distinguish between malignant and benign change in lymph nodes. Lymph nodes with a maximum short diameter of no more than 10 mm are generally accepted as benign. However, this criterion has 2 main limitations: the proportion of nodes that harbor metastases from urogenital cancers is usually smaller; and nodal hyperplasia also can cause volume increase of lymph nodes.[4,5] When using a common size standard of 10 mm, a high false-negative rate caused by the involved nodes of normal size may weaken the diagnostic accuracy of lymph node metastasis on MR imaging in patients with prostate cancers. If the size standard decreases to 6 mm, a higher sensitivity (78%) and specificity (98%) can be obtained.[19] Hence, some investigators have proposed that the size criterion should be altered according to the location of the node and the primary tumor. Grubnic and colleagues[20] advocate that lymph nodes with a maximum short-axis diameter of more than 6 mm in the pelvis and 5 mm in the retroperitoneum should be considered abnormal. Vinnicombe and colleagues[21] suggested that the upper limit of the maximum short-axis diameter for normal lymph nodes in patients with testicular tumors should be 10 mm for the external iliac region, 9 mm for the common iliac region, and 7 mm for the internal iliac region. Koh and colleagues[22] suggested a maximum short-axis diameter of 8 mm in patients with testicular cancer for retroperitoneal lymph nodes. Gualdi and colleagues[23] and Brown and colleagues[24] suggested that lymph node size was not a useful criterion. Thin-slice MR imaging of 3-mm to 4-mm slice interval and 0.4-mm to 0.5-mm interslice gap could detect a larger number of lymph nodes than a 5-mm slice interval and 3-mm interslice gap, suggesting the importance of protocol selection in the

Table 2
Secondary features to distinguish benign from malignant lymph nodes

Criteria	Benign	Malignant
Shape	Ovoid or elongated	Round or spherical
Conture	Smooth	Irregular/lobulated/speculated
Signal abnormality	Homogenous on T2WI	Heterogeneous on T2WI
Necrosis	Necrosis (in tuberculosis, fungal infection and cavitating node syndrome, after therapy)	Central necrosis
Fatty hilum	Preserved	Loss
Enhancement	Homogeneous	Heterogeneous, similar to the primary tumor
Location	Scattered distribution	Clustered distribution

Abbreviation: T2WI, T2-weighted imaging.

clarification of metastasis. In rectal cancer, for instance, MR imaging is able to detect perirectal and presacral lymph nodes with sizes ranging from 1 to 5 mm.[25]

Shape and contour of the nodes

Shape and contour of the nodes can be useful in the distinction of metastasis from benign nodes. Most benign nodes are ovoid, as opposed to malignant nodes, which tend to have a rounded shape, although combining the criteria of size and shape does not improve the accuracy of radiological assessment of urogenital pelvic cancers compared with using size as the single criterion. Nodal involvement might lead to an irregular node border if extracapsular extension of metastatic disease is present (**Fig. 6**), although this sign is rarely observed in small nodal metastases.[5,26]

Signal abnormalities

Signal abnormalities of involved lymph nodes are mainly caused by altered nodal composition caused by tumor deposits. Metastatic nodes show low signal intensity that is usually a little higher than that of normal vessels on T1-weighted images and intermediate signal intensity on T2-weighted images. However, signal intensities of malignant nodes often do not differ from those of benign nodes on T1-weighted and T2-weighted images because T1 and T2 relaxation times of metastatic and normal nodes overlap considerably.[27] Heterogeneous signal inside nodes on T2-weighted images, especially necrosis, is more likely to be malignant than homogeneous nodes (**Fig. 6**).[14] Internal abnormalities such as loss of fatty hilum, calcifications and accumulations of fat or fluid may be helpful for identifying nodal metastases, which may resemble a primary malignancy in the signal intensity on MR imaging.

Nodal calcifications may be seen in metastasis from bladder cancer, although it is not a reliable sign because it can also be seen in benign inflammatory disease such as tuberculosis.[4] Cystic appearance resulting from central necrosis is observed in metastatic nodes, especially from the testicular nonseminomatous germ cell tumors, which have high signal intensity on T2-weighted images. Noncystic but large metastatic nodes can appear heterogeneous, with a central low-density component that can be caused by necrosis, but this finding can also be seen in tuberculosis and various fungal infections. Such a central zone of necrosis is only rarely found in metastatic retroperitoneal and pelvic nodes.[28–30] This finding can be further shown by administration of contrast agents. Inhomogeneous enhancement with an enlarged size or similar enhancement with primary tumor strongly implies malignant infiltration in nodes. Moreover, on enhanced scan, a signal intensity time curve may be helpful for detecting nodal involvement in normal-sized nodes.[31]

Location of lymph node

The location of lymph nodes can aid in resolving the ambiguities regarding the metastasis. Nodes that are located along the pathway of lymphatic drainage from a primary tumor, when borderline in size or when they have had a recent increase in size, are more likely to contain metastatic infiltration. The distribution of cluster nodes, even normal-sized nodes, is also considered suspicious for metastasis.[32]

METASTASES TO PELVIC ORGANS
Prostate

Primary prostate cancer is one of the most common malignancies likely to metastasize, whereas

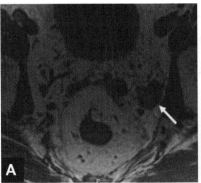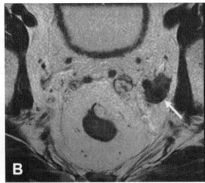

Fig. 6. Pathologically proven metastatic lymph node in a 60-year-old man with rectal cancer. (*A*) Axial T1-weighted image shows lobular left internal iliac lymph node (*arrow*) with heterogeneous signal and loss of central fatty hilum, suspicious of malignant lymph node. (*B*) On axial T2-weighted image it shows heterogeneous signal intensity within (*arrow*).

metastatic malignancy of the prostate is extremely rare. Secondary neoplasms of prostate only account for 0.5% to 5.6% of patients and represent 2.1% of all prostate tumors.[33] The most common primary sites for metastases to the prostate are the lung and pancreas.[34–36] MR imaging is the most valuable imaging method for prostate tumors at present. It can provide precise anatomic information and better characterization of lesions.

Penis

Metastatic penile lesions are extremely rare. Common sites of primary tumors include the urinary bladder (in 30%–35% of cases), the prostate (in 28%–30%), the rectosigmoid colon (in 13%), the kidneys (in 8%–10%), and the testes (in 5%).[37] Penile metastasis signifies advanced disease and poor prognosis. Most metastatic tumors are located in the middle to distal portion of the shaft. Although penile masses are easy to detect by clinical examination, imaging methods are better in the assessment of tumor invasion and discovery of nonpalpable lesions. MR imaging shows higher accuracy in their diagnosis compared with ultrasonography or computed tomography (CT) scans. The common signs of metastatic lesions are ill-defined discrete masses located mostly within the corpora cavernosa, with low signal intensity on T1-weighted imaging (T1WI) and heterogeneous signal intensity on T2-weighted imaging (T2WI). Sagittal images offer visualization of the penile urethra along its length, thereby aiding detection of any obstructing/impinging lesions (**Fig. 7**).[38,39]

Testis

Apart from lymphoma and leukemia, secondary testicular tumors are rare, with an incidence of 0.02% to 2.5% on autopsy.[40] The most common primary site is the prostate, followed by the lung, gastrointestinal tract, melanoma, and kidney. Metastatic lesions tend to appear in unilateral testis and bilateral involvement is seen only in about 15% of cases.[41] Imaging plays an important role in the assessment of metastases to testis. Metastatic lesions are always seen as ill-defined, heterogeneous, solid masses. MR imaging of the scrotum is an efficient imaging tool in detecting metastatic masses when sonographic findings are inconclusive, especially in cases in which the scrotum is markedly enlarged. The technique is also helpful for differentiating intratesticular masses from extratesticular masses and provides more anatomic and morphologic information for intratesticular masses.[42] Multinodular intratesticular lesion of mainly low signal intensity on T2WI or an inhomogeneous mass with variable signal intensity on T2WI are considered suggestive of malignant testicular tumors. Heterogeneous enhancement and necrosis are also concerning for malignant features.[43,44] However, these signs are not specific for secondary testicular tumors.

Bladder

Secondary bladder tumors from a distant organ are rare and represent no more than 3% of all malignant bladder tumors. The most common distant metastasizing tumors are breast, followed by melanoma and gastric carcinoma.[45] Adenocarcinoma is the most common histologic type of secondary bladder neoplasms.[46] Most metastatic tumors present in imaging studies as one or multiple mural masses projecting into the bladder lumen. However, in some cases diffuse thickening of the bladder wall can be observed. The high soft tissue contrast of MR imaging permits distinction of

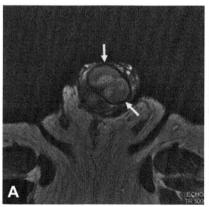
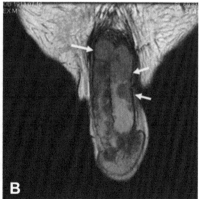

Fig. 7. A 95-year-old man with a history of prostate cancer and penile metastasis. (A) Axial T2-weighted image and (B) coronal T2-weighted image show heterogeneous signal intensity areas of metastatic deposits (arrows) in the corpus spongiosum and cavernosum.

bladder wall layers. T1-weighted images with high contrast between tumor and peribladder fat are optimal for detection of extravesical infiltration, and T2-weighted images with good contrast between tumor and muscle layers of the bladder wall are optimal for evaluation of invaded depth and for differentiating tumor from fibrosis.[47] In addition, bladder distension and sagittal or coronal imaging are used to find small mural nodules, masses, or mural thickening as signs of metastatic involvement of the bladder.

Rectum

Metastatic tumors of the gastrointestinal tract are unusual, especially in the rectum.[48] The common primary tumors include breast cancer, melanoma, ovary, and bladder.[49] In most cases, metastatic lesions of the rectum are seen as asymmetric circumferential thickening of the rectal wall with significant enhancement.[48,50,51] MR imaging, especially with high-resolution sequences and endorectal coils, can accurately delineate the extent of rectal tumors, depth of tumor invasion, relationship to mesorectal fascia, and extramural vascular invasion.[52] Sagittal T2WI is obtained mainly for tumor location and assessment of the relationship between the tumor and the peritoneal reflection; axial images of the tumor are used to reduce the overestimation of the tumor depth of invasion noted on oblique imaging; coronal images are beneficial for identifying the relationship of low rectal tumors to the sphincter.[52,53]

PERITONEAL METASTASIS

Parietal peritoneum lines the pelvic sidewalls and reflects over the bladder and rectum. The inferior extent of the pelvic peritoneal reflections forms the rectovesicle pouch in men. The dome of the bladder is also covered by peritoneum. The rectovesicle pouch or rectouterine pouch is the first site to accumulate ascitic fluid in the pelvis. Disseminated tumors commonly seed these pelvic recesses, followed by accumulation of increasing amounts of ascites in the bilateral paravesical recesses.[54] Tumor involving the PSWs may manifest as slight thickening and enhancement of the sidewall peritoneum. Maximal distension of small bowel and colon with intraluminal contrast material is required for the imaging of peritoneal tumor involving the bowel serosa. Small peritoneal tumors (<1 cm) or diffuse carcinomatosis are difficult to display on unenhanced MR images, but moderate-sized and large peritoneal masses can be visualized on fat-suppressed T2-weighted images as heterogeneous peritoneal masses with intermediate signal intensity. Peritoneal and serosal tumors are displayed as areas of high signal intensity in the setting of diffuse carcinomatosis with ascites. Ascites and most bowel contents are suppressed on diffusion-weighted images, increasing the conspicuity of the adjacent peritoneal tumors.[54–57]

Peritoneal tumors typically enhance slowly with gadolinium and are best visualized on images obtained 5 to 10 minutes after injection of gadolinium chelates. Compared with enhanced CT, gadolinium-enhanced MR is more sensitive to distinguish small enhancing peritoneal tumors from ascites in the pelvis. In a study by Low and colleagues,[54] the sensitivity of images for depicting peritoneal tumors less than 1 cm was as high as 85% to 90%, compared with 22% to 33% for CT. The overall sensitivity of MR imaging in detecting peritoneal tumors of all sizes is as high as 84%,[58] and as low as 54% for CT.[54] Peritoneal tumors can vary from large tumor masses to a thin line of peritoneum with abnormal moderate to marked enhancement (**Fig. 8**), whereas ascites

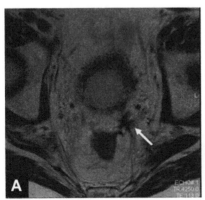
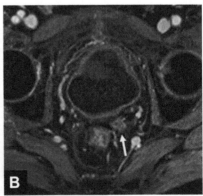

Fig. 8. An 81-year-old man with a history of prostate cancer and pelvic peritoneal metastasis. (A) Axial T2-weighted image shows irregular low signal intensity soft tissue nodule (*arrow*) at left mesorectal fascia. (B) On enhanced T1-weighted postcontrast image, the nodule (*arrow*) shows significant enhancement.

does not enhance. Small enhancing peritoneal tumors may show high signal intensity on the corresponding fat-suppressed T2-weighted images. Inflammatory and malignant disease of the peritoneum can have an identical appearance; for instance, peritonitis and peritoneal carcinomatosis both have delayed enhancement with intravenous gadolinium.[55,56]

Pseudomyxoma Peritonei Syndrome

Pseudomyxoma peritonei syndrome (PMP) is a special type of peritoneal metastasis that is commonly secondary to mucinous malignancies of appendix and ovary. PMP features the accumulation of gelatinous tumor exudate throughout the peritoneal cavity, resulting from escape of mucin-producing tumor cells from appendix or ovary and spreading in the peritoneal cavity. The peritoneal tumors in this condition are best staged and characterized by delayed gadolinium-enhanced MR imaging with fat suppression. The contrast resolution of MR aids in distinguishing nonenhancing ascites and mucin from the cellular component of pseudomyxoma peritonei, which enhances with contrast medium, as opposed to ascites or mucin, which do not show any enhancement with gadolinium (**Fig. 9**). Solid adenocarcinoma shows marked enhancement, whereas adenocarcinoma mixed with mucin shows mild to moderate enhancement.[59]

METASTASIS TO SKELETAL MUSCLE

Metastases in skeletal musculature are rare, with prevalences ranging from 0.03% to 5.6% in autopsy and from 1.2% to 1.8% in radiological series.[60] According to the diverse features of skeletal muscle metastases (SMMs) on CT, Surov and colleagues[61,62] classified them into 5 different types: type I, focal intramuscular masses with homogeneous contrast enhancement; type II, abscesslike intramuscular lesions (**Fig. 10**); type III, diffuse metastatic muscle infiltration; type IV, multifocal intramuscular calcification; type V, intramuscular bleeding. The largest proportion of SMMs presents as intramuscular masses, mostly as a single mass. These masses can be isointense compared with the unaffected muscle tissue on T1WI and hyperintense on T2-weighted images with or without fat saturation with the exception of melanoma, pulmonary angiosarcoma, and adrenal cell carcinoma metastasis, which are typically hyperintense on T1WI. These hyperintense intramuscular metastases on T1 images can mimic benign muscle lesions, such as lipoma or hemangioma or intramuscular bleeding. Postcontrast T1-weighted images aid in this differential diagnosis.[61,63] After administration of contrast medium, most muscle metastases, especially those associated with necrosis, show marked heterogeneous enhancement, typically extensive peritumoral enhancement. In contrast with other muscle malignancies (ie, muscle lymphomas or sarcomas), most metastatic lesions show well-defined margins, which makes differentiation from benign muscle lesions difficult (eg, focal myositis).[61,63]

BONE METASTASIS

Metastatic lesions are the most common malignancy observed in the skeleton, including the pelvis. About 80% of skeletal metastases come from prostate, lung, breast, and thyroid carcinomas (**Table 3**). Most metastases from the pelvis are from prostate, lung, breast, renal,

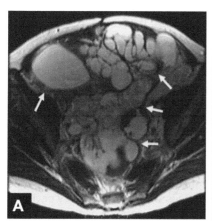 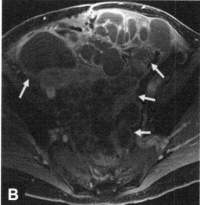

Fig. 9. A 63-year-old man with extensive pseudomyxoma peritonei. (*A*) Axial T2-weighted image shows multiloculated cystic masses in pelvis and lower abdomen (*arrows*). (*B*) Contrast-enhanced axial T1-weighted image shows wall enhancement of the multiloculated cystic masses (*arrows*).

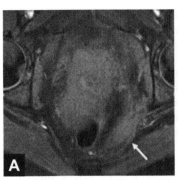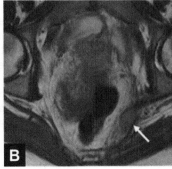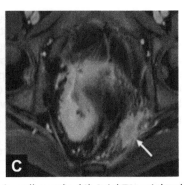

Fig. 10. A 44-year-old man with bladder cancer and metastasis to left pelvic wall muscle. (*A*) Axial T1-weighted image shows infiltrating lesion with isointense signal at left posterior pelvis and piriformis muscle (*arrow*). (*B*) On T2-weighted image the lesion (*arrow*) shows slightly higher signal intensity than on T1WI. (*C*) Contrast-enhanced T1-weighted image shows peripheral enhancement of the lesion (*arrow*).

gastrointestinal, and thyroid carcinomas.[64] The pelvis is the second most common site of bone metastases after the spine, and the sacrum is the most common site of metastasis in the pelvis.[65,66] Most metastatic lesions in the sacrum result from hematogenous spread; however, rectal carcinoma can directly invade the sacrum.[64] Bone metastatic lesions can be osteoblastic (**Fig. 11**), osteolytic (**Fig. 12**), or mixed, but osteolytic lesions are most common (**Table 4**).[64,67,68] Metastatic lesions in multiple myeloma are purely osteolytic. Breast cancer metastasis usually manifests as an osteolytic lesion with reactive osteogenesis. In contrast, prostate cancer manifests as osteoblastic lesions with increased osteoclast activity.[69,70]

Because MR imaging is sensitive for detecting early changes in bone marrow before osteoblastic

response, it is considered the appropriate choice for evaluating early bone metastasis in patients with prostate cancer. Visualization of these metastatic lesions could be improved by T2-weighted fat-suppressed sequences like short T1 inversion recovery (STIR).[64,71,72] Because bone marrow metastasis has signal intensity equal to the primary tumor, it is best recognized on T1-weighted images, which can provide good contrast resolution between metastases and fatty bone marrow. Metastases to the bone marrow show low signal intensity corresponding with a longer T1 relaxation time compared with the high signal intensity of the fatty tissue.[73] On the T2-weighted images, relaxation time lengthens with a significant increase in the metastatic lesions, whereas intermediate signal intensity is observed with the cell-rich tumors. The accompanying osteoblastic component and bone regeneration cause a decrease in the T2 relaxation time and lead to diminished signal intensity on T2-weighted images, which should be supplemented with fat-suppression sequences such as STIR or fat-suppressed T2-weighted sequences. If a lesion is characterized as a halo of high signal intensity surrounding a low-signal lesion in T2WI, as occurs in osteoblastic metastasis, a central part with low signal intensity correlates with the osteoblastic tumor areas, and the high-signal portion of the lesion indicates a perifocal edema. If an edema halo is present, osteoblastic metastases can easily be differentiated from a bone island.[74] Even in massive bone marrow involvement by metastasis, insignificant trabecular bone destruction is observed, which makes bone scans negative, most obvious in bones with large medullary cavities like the vertebral body. In addition, tumor cells positioned between trabeculae cannot be seen on plain-film bone scans, whereas these lesions are easily visualized by MR imaging.[69,71,73]

Table 3
Radiological presentation of bone metastatic from different primary tumors

Primary Organ	Lytic (%)	Mixed (%)	Blastic (%)
Breast	80	10	10
Lung	75	20	5
Stomach	90	10	0
Pancreas	80	10	10
Urinary bladder	90	10	0
Prostate	10	10	80
Colon or rectum	75	5	20
Testis	75	5	20
Malignant melanoma	90	10	0
Carcinoid	5	15	80

Data from Yochum TR, Rowe LJ. Yochum and Rowe's essentials of skeletal radiology. 3rd edition. Baltimore (MD): Lippincott Williams & Wilkins; 2005.

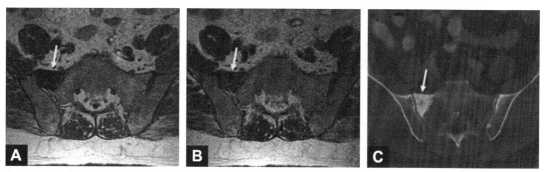

Fig. 11. Osteoblastic bony metastasis in a 70-year-old man with prostate cancer. (*A*) Axial T1-weighted image and (*B*) axial T2-weighted image both showing low signal intensity abnormality (*arrow*) involving the marrow of right sacral ala. (*C*) Bone window CT scan shows sclerotic bony lesion (*arrow*) involving the right sacral ala.

MR imaging has shown increased sensitivity and specificity compared with bone scintigraphy in visualizing bone metastasis (100% vs 46% for sensitivity and 88% vs 32% for specificity). MR imaging can detect bone metastasis in 37.5% of patients with negative plain film and bone scintigraphy.[67,75]

Normal bone marrow has a high-intensity signal on T1 imaging; metastatic lesions show a reduced signal as a result of the replacement of fat in the marrow by the tumor. MR imaging has better contrast resolution than CT for visualizing soft tissue and spinal cord, which is an advantage for distinguishing benign from malignant vertebral compression fractures and spinal cord compression. Bone destruction is more easily detected on radiographs and CT than MR imaging because cortical bone appears hypointense on both T1-weighted and T2-weighted sequences.[76,77] MR imaging can acquire sagittal images of the

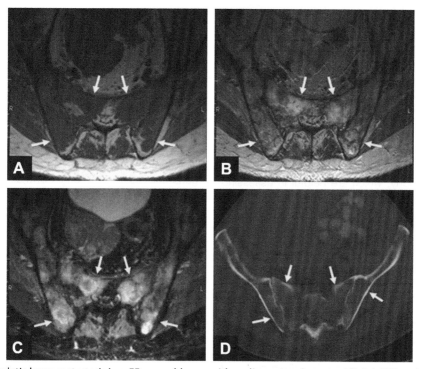

Fig. 12. Osteolytic bony metastasis in a 55-year-old man with malignant melanoma. (*A*) Axial T1-weighted image shows multiple low signal intensity lesions (*arrows*) involving the sacrum and iliac bones. (*B*) On axial T2-weighted image these lesions (*arrows*) show high signal intensity. (*C*) On enhanced T1-weighted image these lesions (*arrows*) show substantial heterogeneous enhancement. (*D*) Axial CT scan in bone window displays their osteoblastic nature (*arrows*).

Table 4
Osteoblastic versus osteoclastic bone metastasis

	T1 Appearance	T2 Appearance
Osteoblastic	Hypointense	T2 relaxation time decreases leading to a diminished signal intensity in T2-weighted images
Osteoclastic	Longer T1 relaxation time (intermediate to hypointense)	Relaxation time lengthens with a significant increase in the signal in the lesion

entire spine, which allows a quick overview of the marrow. Use of contrast-enhanced MR imaging allows distinction between necrotic lesions and progressive lesions and provides adequate information for assessing the treatment response.[78,79]

NEW IMAGING ADVANCES
Diffusion-weighted Imaging and Diffusion-weighted Whole-body Imaging with Background Body Signal Suppression

Diffusion-weighted imaging (DWI) depicts movements of water molecules within the tissues. Increased cellularity as seen in metastatic lesions exhibit restricted diffusion. DWI is used to evaluate the response of primary tumor and metastases to chemotherapy or radiation therapy, by monitoring changes in tumor size and apparent diffusion coefficient values following treatment. It is an excellent tool in the evaluation of lymphadenopathy in patients with predominantly nodal metastasis and lymphoma. The highly cellular lymph nodes are depicted with high tumor-to-background tissue contrast. Even small nodes are easily depicted. However, DWI is prone to motion artifacts. Whole-body diffusion-weighted sequences can generate images similar to those of positron emission tomography, which are helpful in assessing treatment response.[80,81]

Nanoparticle-enhanced MR Imaging

Lymphotrophic nanoparticle–enhanced MR (LNMR) imaging represents one of the most promising functional imaging approaches in the detection of lymph node metastases in patients with cancers. Lymphotropic superparamagnetic ultrasmall particles of iron oxide (USPIO), such as ferumoxytol, are transported through the vascular endothelium into the interstitial space and subsequently via lymph vessels to the lymph nodes. If lymph node regions contain malignant tissue, the absence of macrophage activity results in the affected lymph nodes appearing hyperintense on T2-weighted images. LNMR imaging with ferumoxtran-10 increases the sensitivity for detecting lymph node metastases from 35% when using conventional MR imaging alone to 90%, and to greater than 90% for specificity.[82] In a large study on intermediate-risk to high-risk prostate cancer, LNMR imaging obtained a sensitivity of 82% and negative predictive value of 96%.[83] False-positive results may be seen in benign conditions such as granulomatous diseases causing necrosis of the lymph nodes, nodal fibrosis, and reactive nodal hyperplasia in which normal macrophages are replaced from the lymph node, leading to abnormal uptake patterns on imaging.[14,84] Two main obstacles for USPIO contrasts are commercial nonavailability and time-consuming interpretation. Combination of USPIO and diffusion-weighted MR imaging improves the staging accuracy of normal-sized lymph nodes in patients with bladder and prostate cancer, and decreases the average time needed for analysis from 80 minutes to 13 minutes.[85–87]

SUMMARY

Metastasis to the pelvic organs poses a particular challenge to oncologists because of the intricacy and complexity of the pelvic anatomy. Pelvic organs can also be the origin of malignancies that can spread locally to adjacent structures such as lymph nodes, which makes the proper staging and treatment of these malignancies dependent on the accurate identification of local pelvic metastasis. The current clinical practice relies on structural imaging techniques. Functional imaging techniques like DWI, and USPIO-MR imaging, seem to be promising tools in achieving better characterization of pelvic metastasis. In peritoneal, lymph node, and muscle metastasis, prior experience and meticulous protocol selection are crucial for the correct diagnosis.

REFERENCES

1. Heiken JP, Lee JK. MR imaging of the pelvis. Radiology 1988;166(1 Pt 1):11–6.

2. Barentsz JO, Engelbrecht MR, Witjes JA, et al. MR imaging of the male pelvis. Eur Radiol 1999;9(9): 1722–36.

3. Di Muzio N, Fodor A, Berardi G, et al. Lymph nodal metastases: diagnosis and treatment. Q J Nucl Med Mol Imaging 2012;56(5):421–9.

4. Paño B, Sebastià C, Buñesch L, et al. Pathways of lymphatic spread in male urogenital pelvic malignancies. Radiographics 2011;31(1):135–60.

5. Hedgire SS, Pargaonkar VK, Elmi A, et al. Pelvic nodal imaging. Radiol Clin North Am 2012;50(6): 1111–25.

6. Daneshmand S, Quek ML, Stein JP, et al. Prognosis of patients with lymph node positive prostate cancer following radical prostatectomy: long-term results. J Urol 2004;172(6 Pt 1):2252–5.

7. Leveridge M, Siemens DR, Morash C. What next? Managing lymph nodes in men with penile cancer. Can Urol Assoc J 2008;2(5):525–31.

8. Edge SB, Compton CC. The American Joint Committee on Cancer. AJCC cancer staging manual and the future of TNM. 7th edition. Ann Surg Oncol 2010;17(6):1471–4.

9. Compton CC. AJCC cancer staging atlas. A companion to the seventh editions of the AJCC cancer staging manual and handbook. 2nd edition. New York: Springer; 2012.

10. Morisawa N, Koyama T, Togashi K. Metastatic lymph nodes in urogenital cancers: contribution of imaging findings. Abdom Imaging 2006;31(5): 620–9.

11. Koh DM, Husband JE. Patterns of recurrence of bladder carcinoma following radical cystectomy. Canc Imag 2003;3:96–100.

12. Abol-Enein H, El-Baz M, Abd El-Hameed MA, et al. Lymph node involvement in patients with bladder cancer treated with radical cystectomy: a pathoanatomical study–a single center experience. J Urol 2004;172(5 Pt 1):1818–21.

13. Barentsz JO, Jager GJ, van Vierzen PB, et al. Staging urinary bladder cancer after transurethral biopsy: value of fast dynamic contrast-enhanced MR imaging. Radiology 1996;201(1):185–93.

14. Saokar A, Islam T, Jantsch M, et al. Detection of lymph nodes in pelvic malignancies with computed tomography and magnetic resonance imaging. Clin Imaging 2010;34(5):361–6.

15. Willett CG, Tepper JE, Cohen AM, et al. Failure patterns following curative resection of colonic carcinoma. Ann Surg 1984;200(6):685–90.

16. Cohen AM, Tremiterra S, Candela F, et al. Prognosis of node-positive colon cancer. Cancer 1991;67(7):1859–61.

17. Shihab OC, Taylor F, Bees N, et al. Relevance of magnetic resonance imaging-detected pelvic sidewall lymph node involvement in rectal cancer. Br J Surg 2011;98(12):1798–804.

18. Jager GJ, Barentsz JO, Oosterhof GO, et al. Pelvic adenopathy in prostatic and urinary bladder carcinoma: MR imaging with a three-dimensional TI-weighted magnetization-prepared-rapid gradient-echo sequence. AJR Am J Roentgenol 1996;167(6): 1503–7.

19. Oyen RH, Van Poppel HP, Ameye FE, et al. Lymph node staging of localized prostatic carcinoma with CT and CT-guided fine-needle aspiration biopsy: prospective study of 285 patients. Radiology 1994;190(2):315–22.

20. Grubnic S, Vinnicombe SJ, Norman AR, et al. MR evaluation of normal retroperitoneal and pelvic lymph nodes. Clin Radiol 2002;57(3):193–200 [discussion: 201–4].

21. Vinnicombe SJ, Norman AR, Nicolson V, et al. Normal pelvic lymph nodes: evaluation with CT after bipedal lymphangiography. Radiology 1995; 194(2):349–55.

22. Koh DM, Hughes M, Husband JE. Cross-sectional imaging of nodal metastases in the abdomen and pelvis. Abdom Imaging 2006;31(6):632–43.

23. Gualdi GF, Casciani E, Guadalaxara A, et al. Local staging of rectal cancer with transrectal ultrasound and endorectal magnetic resonance imaging: comparison with histologic findings. Dis Colon Rectum 2000;43(3):338–45.

24. Brown G, Radcliffe AG, Newcombe RG, et al. Preoperative assessment of prognostic factors in rectal cancer using high-resolution magnetic resonance imaging. Br J Surg 2003;90(3):355–64.

25. Matsuoka H, Nakamura A, Sugiyama M, et al. MRI diagnosis of mesorectal lymph node metastasis in patients with rectal carcinoma. What is the optimal criterion? Anticancer Res 2004;24(6):4097–101.

26. Bellin MF, Lebleu L, Meric JB. Evaluation of retroperitoneal and pelvic lymph node metastases with MRI and MR lymphangiography. Abdom Imaging 2003;28(2):155–63.

27. Dooms GC, Hricak H, Moseley ME, et al. Characterization of lymphadenopathy by magnetic resonance relaxation times: preliminary results. Radiology 1985;155(3):691–7.

28. Hulnick DH, Megibow AJ, Naidich DP, et al. Abdominal tuberculosis: CT evaluation. Radiology 1985;157(1):199–204.

29. Huppert BJ, Farrell MA. Case 60: cavitating mesenteric lymph node syndrome. Radiology 2003;228(1):180–4.

30. Krishnam MS, Suh RD, Tomasian A, et al. Postoperative complications of lung transplantation: radiologic findings along a time continuum. Radiographics 2007;27(4):957–74.

31. Noworolski SM, Fischbein NJ, Kaplan MJ, et al. Challenges in dynamic contrast-enhanced MRI imaging of cervical lymph nodes to detect metastatic disease. J Magn Reson Imaging 2003;17(4):455–62.

32. Roy C, Le Bras Y, Mangold L, et al. Small pelvic lymph node metastases: evaluation with MR imaging. Clin Radiol 1997;52(6):437–40.

33. Balaban M, Selimoglu A, Horuz R, et al. Prostate metastasis of malignant melanoma. Korean J Urol 2013;54(7):486–9.

34. Bates AW, Baithun SI. Secondary solid neoplasms of the prostate: a clinico-pathological series of 51 cases. Virchows Arch 2002;440(4):392–6.

35. Claus FG, Hricak H, Hattery RR. Pretreatment evaluation of prostate cancer: role of MR imaging and 1H MR spectroscopy. Radiographics 2004; 24(Suppl 1):S167–80.

36. Scheidler J, Hricak H, Vigneron DB, et al. Prostate cancer: localization with three-dimensional proton MR spectroscopic imaging–clinicopathologic study. Radiology 1999;213(2):473–80.

37. Berger AP, Rogatsch H, Hoeltl L, et al. Late penile metastasis from primary bladder carcinoma. Urology 2003;62(1):145.

38. Lau TN, Wakeley CJ, Goddard P. Magnetic resonance imaging of penile metastases: a report on five cases. Australas Radiol 1999;43(3):378–81.

39. Hricak H, Marotti M, Gilbert TJ, et al. Normal penile anatomy and abnormal penile conditions: evaluation with MR imaging. Radiology 1988;169(3):683–90.

40. Marble EJ. Testicular metastasis from carcinoma of the prostate: review of literature and report of a case. J Urol 1960;84:369–75.

41. Haupt HM, Mann RB, Trump DL, et al. Metastatic carcinoma involving the testis. Clinical and pathologic distinction from primary testicular neoplasms. Cancer 1984;54(4):709–14.

42. Tsili AC, Argyropoulou MI, Giannakis D, et al. MRI in the characterization and local staging of testicular neoplasms. AJR Am J Roentgenol 2010; 194(3):682–9.

43. Johnson JO, Mattrey RF, Phillipson J. Differentiation of seminomatous from nonseminomatous testicular tumors with MR imaging. AJR Am J Roentgenol 1990;154(3):539–43.

44. Tsili AC, Tsampoulas C, Giannakopoulos X, et al. MRI in the histologic characterization of testicular neoplasms. AJR Am J Roentgenol 2007;189(6): W331–7.

45. Morichetti D, Mazzucchelli R, Lopez-Beltran A, et al. Secondary neoplasms of the urinary system and male genital organs. BJU Int 2009;104(6):770–6.

46. Wong-You-Cheong JJ, Woodward PJ, Manning MA, et al. From the Archives of the AFIP: neoplasms of the urinary bladder: radiologic-pathologic correlation. Radiographics 2006;26(2):553–80.

47. Barentsz JO, Witjes JA, Ruijs JH. What is new in bladder cancer imaging. Urol Clin North Am 1997;24(3):583–602.

48. Bamias A, Baltayiannis G, Kamina S, et al. Rectal metastases from lobular carcinoma of the breast: report of a case and literature review. Ann Oncol 2001;12(5):715–8.

49. Washington K, McDonagh D. Secondary tumors of the gastrointestinal tract: surgical pathologic findings and comparison with autopsy survey. Mod Pathol 1995;8(4):427–33.

50. Venara A, Thibaudeau E, Lebdai S, et al. Rectal metastasis of prostate cancer: about a case. J Clin Med Res 2010;2(3):137–9.

51. Saranovic D, Kovac JD, Knezevic S, et al. Invasive lobular breast cancer presenting an unusual metastatic pattern in the form of peritoneal and rectal metastases: a case report. J Breast Cancer 2011; 14(3):247–50.

52. Gowdra Halappa V, Corona Villalobos CP, Bonekamp S, et al. Rectal imaging: part 1, High-resolution MRI of carcinoma of the rectum at 3 T. AJR Am J Roentgenol 2012;199(1): W35–42.

53. Brown G, Richards CJ, Newcombe RG, et al. Rectal carcinoma: thin-section MR imaging for staging in 28 patients. Radiology 1999;211(1):215–22.

54. Low RN, Sigeti JS. MR imaging of peritoneal disease: comparison of contrast-enhanced fast multiplanar spoiled gradient-recalled and spin-echo imaging. AJR Am J Roentgenol 1994;163(5):1131–40.

55. Low RN, Barone RM, Lacey C, et al. Peritoneal tumor: MR imaging with dilute oral barium and intravenous gadolinium-containing contrast agents compared with unenhanced MR imaging and CT. Radiology 1997;204(2):513–20.

56. Low RN. Gadolinium-enhanced MR imaging of liver capsule and peritoneum. Magn Reson Imaging Clin N Am 2001;9(4):803–19, vii.

57. Low RN. MR imaging of the peritoneal spread of malignancy. Abdom Imaging 2007;32(3):267–83.

58. Low RN, Barone RM, Gurney JM, et al. Mucinous appendiceal neoplasms: preoperative MR staging and classification compared with surgical and histopathologic findings. AJR Am J Roentgenol 2008; 190(3):656–65.

59. Szklaruk J, Tamm EP, Choi H, et al. MR imaging of common and uncommon large pelvic masses. Radiographics 2003;23(2):403–24.

60. Surov A, Pawelka MK, Wienke A, et al. PET/CT imaging of skeletal muscle metastases. Acta Radiol 2014;55(1):101–6.

61. Surov A, Fiedler E, Voigt W, et al. Magnetic resonance imaging of intramuscular metastases. Skeletal Radiol 2011;40(4):439–46.

62. Surov A, Hainz M, Holzhausen HJ, et al. Skeletal muscle metastases: primary tumours, prevalence, and radiological features. Eur Radiol 2010;20(3): 649–58.

63. Arpaci T, Ugurluer G, Akbas T, et al. Imaging of the skeletal muscle metastases. Eur Rev Med Pharmacol Sci 2012;16(15):2057–63.

64. Messiou C, Cook G, deSouza NM. Imaging metastatic bone disease from carcinoma of the prostate. Br J Cancer 2009;101(8):1225–32.

65. Coleman RE. Metastatic bone disease: clinical features, pathophysiology and treatment strategies. Cancer Treat Rev 2001;27(3):165–76.

66. Papagelopoulos PJ, Savvidou OD, Galanis EC, et al. Advances and challenges in diagnosis and management of skeletal metastases. Orthopedics 2006;29(7):609–20 [quiz: 621–2].

67. Lecouvet FE, Geukens D, Stainier A, et al. Magnetic resonance imaging of the axial skeleton for detecting bone metastases in patients with high-risk prostate cancer: diagnostic and cost-effectiveness and comparison with current detection strategies. J Clin Oncol 2007;25(22):3281–7.

68. Disler DG, Miklic D. Imaging findings in tumors of the sacrum. AJR Am J Roentgenol 1999;173(6): 1699–706.

69. Taoka T, Mayr NA, Lee HJ, et al. Factors influencing visualization of vertebral metastases on MR imaging versus bone scintigraphy. AJR Am J Roentgenol 2001;176(6):1525–30.

70. Roodman GD. Mechanisms of bone metastasis. N Engl J Med 2004;350(16):1655–64.

71. Yamaguchi T, Tamai K, Yamato M, et al. Intertrabecular pattern of tumors metastatic to bone. Cancer 1996;78(7):1388–94.

72. Pearce T, Philip S, Brown J, et al. Bone metastases from prostate, breast and multiple myeloma: differences in lesion conspicuity at short-tau inversion recovery and diffusion-weighted MRI. Br J Radiol 2012;85(1016):1102–6.

73. Algra PR, Bloem JL, Tissing H, et al. Detection of vertebral metastases: comparison between MR imaging and bone scintigraphy. Radiographics 1991; 11(2):219–32.

74. Schweitzer ME, Levine C, Mitchell DG, et al. Bull's-eyes and halos: useful MR discriminators of osseous metastases. Radiology 1993;188(1): 249–52.

75. Wang CK, Li CW, Hsieh TJ, et al. Characterization of bone and soft-tissue tumors with in vivo 1H MR spectroscopy: initial results. Radiology 2004; 232(2):599–605.

76. Simpfendorfer CS, Ilaslan H, Davies AM, et al. Does the presence of focal normal marrow fat signal within a tumor on MRI exclude malignancy? An analysis of 184 histologically proven tumors of the pelvic and appendicular skeleton. Skeletal Radiol 2008;37(9):797–804.

77. Ghanem N, Uhl M, Brink I, et al. Diagnostic value of MRI in comparison to scintigraphy, PET, MS-CT and PET/CT for the detection of metastases of bone. Eur J Radiol 2005;55(1):41–55.

78. Schmidt GP, Reiser MF, Baur-Melnyk A. Whole-body MRI for the staging and follow-up of patients with metastasis. Eur J Radiol 2009;70(3):393–400.

79. Schmidt GP, Schoenberg SO, Reiser MF, et al. Whole-body MR imaging of bone marrow. Eur J Radiol 2005;55(1):33–40.

80. Kwee TC, Takahara T, Luijten PR, et al. ADC measurements of lymph nodes: inter- and intra-observer reproducibility study and an overview of the literature. Eur J Radiol 2010;75(2):215–20.

81. Low RN. Diffusion-weighted MR imaging for whole body metastatic disease and lymphadenopathy. Magn Reson Imaging Clin N Am 2009;17(2):245–61.

82. Harisinghani MG, Barentsz J, Hahn PF, et al. Noninvasive detection of clinically occult lymph-node metastases in prostate cancer. N Engl J Med 2003;348(25):2491–9.

83. Heesakkers RA, Hövels AM, Jager GJ, et al. MRI with a lymph-node-specific contrast agent as an alternative to CT scan and lymph-node dissection in patients with prostate cancer: a prospective multicohort study. Lancet Oncol 2008;9(9):850–6.

84. Talab SS, Preston MA, Elmi A, et al. Prostate cancer imaging: what the urologist wants to know. Radiol Clin North Am 2012;50(6):1015–41.

85. Briganti A. How to improve the ability to detect pelvic lymph node metastases of urologic malignancies. Eur Urol 2009;55(4):770–2.

86. Deserno WM, Harisinghani MG, Taupitz M, et al. Urinary bladder cancer: preoperative nodal staging with ferumoxtran-10-enhanced MR imaging. Radiology 2004;233(2):449–56.

87. Mattei A, Danuser H. Contemporary imaging analyses of pelvic lymph nodes in the prostate cancer patient. Curr Opin Urol 2011;21(3):211–8.

MR Imaging of Scrotum

Athina C. Tsili, MD[a],*, Dimitrios Giannakis, MD[b],
Anastasios Sylakos, MD[b], Alexandra Ntorkou, MD[c],
Nikolaos Sofikitis, MD[b], Maria I. Argyropoulou, MD[a]

KEYWORDS

- Magnetic resonance • Imaging • Testis • Scrotum • Testicular carcinoma

KEY POINTS

- Magnetic resonance (MR) imaging of the scrotum represents a valuable supplemental diagnostic tool in the investigation of scrotal diseases.
- The technique is particularly recommended in cases of inconclusive or nondiagnostic sonographic findings.
- MR imaging of the scrotum with respect to lesion location, morphology, and tissue characterization provides important information in the presurgical work-up of scrotal masses, improving patient care and decreasing the number of unnecessary surgical explorations.
- The technique performs well in the localization of a scrotal mass, in the differentiation of paratesticular masses, in the distinction between benign from malignant intratesticular lesions, and in the evaluation of the local extent of the disease in cases of testicular carcinomas.

INTRODUCTION

Imaging has an important role in the investigation of scrotal diseases, although clinical examination represents the primary method for the evaluation of scrotal abnormalities. Sonography currently remains the modality of choice in the initial assessment of scrotal lesions.[1–8] It is easily performed, widely available, inexpensive, and has been shown to be highly sensitive in the identification of scrotal masses.[1–8] However, a confident characterization of the nature of intratesticular and paratesticular masses is not always possible, based on sonographic findings only. Magnetic resonance (MR) imaging of the scrotum has been proposed as an alternative imaging technique for the evaluation of scrotal diseases.[9–42] It is a useful diagnostic tool for the morphologic assessment and tissue characterization in the work-up of scrotal masses and reduces the need for diagnostic surgical explorations of the scrotum. The advantages of MR imaging include simultaneous imaging of both testicles, paratesticular spaces, and spermatic cords; adequate anatomic information; satisfactory tissue contrast; and functional information.[9–42] MR imaging may be a valuable problem-solving tool in the assessment of scrotal diseases when sonographic findings are equivocal or inconsistent with the clinical findings. Serra and colleagues[16] reported that MR imaging of the scrotum, when performed after inconclusive ultrasound examination, may be diagnostic and cost-effective, although in this study it was required only in 1.4% of cases.

Determining the accurate location of a scrotal mass, whether intratesticular or paratesticular, is important to ensure adequate treatment planning. Most paratesticular masses are benign; therefore,

Competing financial interests: The authors declare that they have no competing financial interests.
[a] Department of Clinical Radiology, Medical School, University of Ioannina, Ioannina 45110, Greece;
[b] Department of Urology, Medical School, University of Ioannina, Ioannina 45110, Greece; [c] Department of Clinical Radiology, University Hospital of Ioannina, Leoforos S. Niarchou, Ioannina 45500, Greece
* Corresponding author. Department of Clinical Radiology, Medical School, University of Ioannina, Ioannina 45110, Greece.
E-mail addresses: a_tsili@yahoo.gr; atsili@cc.uoi.gr

Magn Reson Imaging Clin N Am 22 (2014) 217–238
http://dx.doi.org/10.1016/j.mric.2014.01.007

mri.theclinics.com

radical orchiectomy may be obviated.[13,14,43–50] MR imaging of the scrotum has been proved highly accurate in the differentiation of extratesticular from intratesticular disease, being superior to sonography especially in cases when the scrotum is markedly enlarged. MR imaging findings with respect to tumor location, morphologic features, and tissue characterization can aid in narrowing the differential diagnosis in cases of paratesticular masses.[13,14,43–50]

Although most intratesticular masses are malignant, a possible diagnosis of various benign intratesticular entities, including dilatation of rete testis, epidermoid cyst, fibrosis, orchitis, infarction, hematoma, and hemorrhagic necrosis, based on MR features may improve patient care and decrease the number of unnecessary radical surgical procedures.[9–12,17,51–57] In these cases, follow-up, lesion biopsy, tumor enucleation, and testis-sparing surgery (TSS) may be justified. MR imaging of the testicles may provide important information in the preoperative characterization of the histologic nature of various intratesticular mass lesions in terms of morphologic information and by showing the presence of fat, fibrous tissue, fluid, and solid contrast-enhancing tissue within the masses.[9–12,17,51–57]

According to the current guidelines, radical orchiectomy remains the treatment of choice for testis neoplasms of malignant and unknown origin.[58–61] Nevertheless, in the last years the management of testicular tumors has started to change in favor of conservative surgery.[58–61] The widespread use of sonography has led to a marked increase in the number of incidentally detected, small-sized testicular mass lesions, most of which have been proved to be benign. TSS has recently been proposed as an alternative option in selected cases, namely, in small malignant germ cell tumors (GCTs) arising in both or in solitary testes, coupled with local adjuvant radiotherapy and in small Leydig cell tumors, with elective indications (healthy contralateral testes), provided that pathology fails to reveal aggressive features.[58–61] TSS is also an option in small sonographically detected, nonpalpable tumors provided that histology excludes malignancy (the incidence of benign pathology is reported at approximately 80% in these cases).[58–61]

Accurate preoperative imaging evaluation of the local stage of disease is mandatory in the care of patients who are candidates for TSS. MR imaging of the scrotum performs well in the evaluation of the local extent of testicular carcinomas.[17] Moreover, MR imaging findings can be closely correlated with the histologic characteristics of testicular neoplasms, providing a preoperative classification of the histologic type of testicular tumors.[18,34]

MR IMAGING PROTOCOL

MR imaging of the scrotum is performed with the use of a pelvic phased array coil or a surface coil. Patients are examined in the supine position, with the testes placed at a similar distance from the coil, usually by means of a towel placed beneath the testis and the penis draped on the anterior abdominal wall.

The MR imaging protocol should include

1. Thin-section spin-echo T1-weighted images in the transverse plane should be included. These images provide information about scrotal anatomy and demonstrate hyperintense lesions.
2. Axial fat-suppressed T1-weighted sequences are repeated when a lesion with high T1 signal intensity is detected.
3. Thin-section fast spin-echo T2-weighted images in 2 or 3 planes should be included, including the transverse plane and the coronal and/or the sagittal plane. These images are best for lesion detection, localization, and characterization. On the coronal plane, a comparative evaluation of both testes, the paratesticular spaces, and the spermatic cords is possible.

Dynamic contrast-enhanced (DCE) subtracted MR imaging, diffusion-weighted imaging (DWI), and MR spectroscopy (MRS) have recently added important diagnostic information in the investigation of scrotal diseases.[62–80] DCE MR imaging provides information regarding the characteristics of microvasculature of testicular carcinomas and assesses tumor angiogenesis.[81–83] In malignancies, DCE MR imaging typically shows rapid and intense enhancement, followed by a relatively rapid washout of the contrast medium; this was also proved for testicular carcinomas.[62–64,81–84] DCE MR imaging has been proved useful in the characterization of scrotal lesions and in the distinction between testicular torsion and trauma from other causes of acute pain.[62–69] DCE MR imaging in combination with T2- and T2*-weighted images is useful in the diagnosis of testicular torsion and in the detection of testicular necrosis.[66] A sensitivity of 100% was referred for DCE-MR imaging in diagnosing complete torsion by showing a decrease or lack of testicular perfusion.[66] The same group of researchers described the differences of testicular enhancement patterns in 42 patients with a variety of scrotal diseases.[63] They concluded that the relative percentages of peak height and mean slope based on time-signal intensity (TSI) curves may be used to differentiate intratesticular from extratesticular diseases.[62] DCE subtracted MR imaging has also been used for the differential diagnosis between benign and malignant intratesticular lesions.[62] The progression of enhancement was classified according to the shape of the TSI curves into 3 types: type I curve, with a linear increase of contrast enhancement over the entire dynamic period, indicating a benign diagnosis; type II curve, with an initial upstroke, after which the signal intensity either plateaus or gradually increases in the late contrast-enhanced period, also suggestive of benignity; and type III curve, with an initial upstroke, followed by gradual washout of the contrast medium, indicating a diagnosis of malignancy (**Fig. 1**). The relative percentages of peak height, maximum time to peak, and mean slope were calculated to assess possible independent predictors of malignancy.[62] A significant association between the type of the TSI curve and the final diagnosis was demonstrated, and the relative percentages of maximum time to peak proved to be the most important discriminating factor in characterizing intratesticular masses.[62]

DWI is an evolving technique that can be used to improve tissue characterization when interpreted in combination with the findings of conventional MR sequences.[84–86] Lesion detection and characterization mainly depends on the extent of tissue cellularity, and increased cellularity is associated with restricted diffusion and reduced apparent diffusion coefficient (ADC) values.[84–86] A few series reported the usefulness of a high b value DWI in the detection and localization of nonpalpable undescended testes in children, when combined with conventional MR imaging data.[71,72] The researchers concluded that hypointensity of testicular parenchyma in these patients detected on all sequences, including DWI, may be related to nonviable testis, therefore, preventing unnecessary surgical procedures.[71,72] Other studies concluded that ADC measurements may be used for the early diagnosis of testicular torsion, without the need of intravenous contrast media, reporting significantly lower mean ADC of the twisted testes than that of the normal contralateral testes because of the presence of ischemia and/or hemorrhagic necrosis.[73,74] DWI and ADC measurements have been reported to be useful in differentiating between normal, benign, and malignant scrotal contents when interpreted in combination with the conventional MR imaging.[87] By combining DWI ($b = 900$ s/mm^2) with conventional MR imaging, an accuracy of 100% has been reported in the characterization of scrotal lesions.[70]

The MR imaging protocol for the evaluation of scrotal masses is described in **Table 1**.

Proton MRS (^{1}H-MRS) provides chemical data on tissue components and has been recently

Table 1 Suggested MR imaging protocol for imaging of the scrotum	
Sequences	**Parameters**
Transverse spin-echo T1-weighted In cases of hyperintense lesions on T1-weighted images, repeated with fat saturation	TR/TE (ms): 500–650/ 13–15 Slice thickness (mm): 3–4 Gap (mm): 0.5 Matrix (mm): 180 × 256 FOV (mm): 240 × 270
Transverse, coronal and sagittal fast-spin echo T2-weighted	TR/TE (ms): 3900/120 Slice thickness (mm): 3–4 Gap (mm): 0.5 Matrix (mm): 180 × 256 FOV (mm): 240 × 270
Transverse DW single-shot, multi-slice spin-echo planar diffusion pulse	TR/TE (ms): 4000/115 Slice thickness (mm): 3–4 Gap (mm): 0.5 Matrix (mm): 180 × 256 FOV (mm): 240 × 270 b value (s/mm^2): 0, 900
Coronal dynamic 3D fast-field subtracted postcontrast	TR/TE (ms): 9/4.1 Slice thickness (mm): 4 Gap (mm): 0 Matrix (mm): 256 × 256 FOV (mm): 219 × 219 Flip angle: 35° Dynamic scans: 7 (every 60 s) Contrast material IV (mL/kg): 0.2

Abbreviations: 3D, 3 dimensional; FOV, field of view; IV, intravenous; TR/TE, time repetition/time echo.

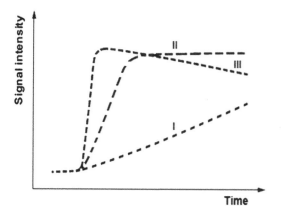

Fig. 1. The TSI curve types.

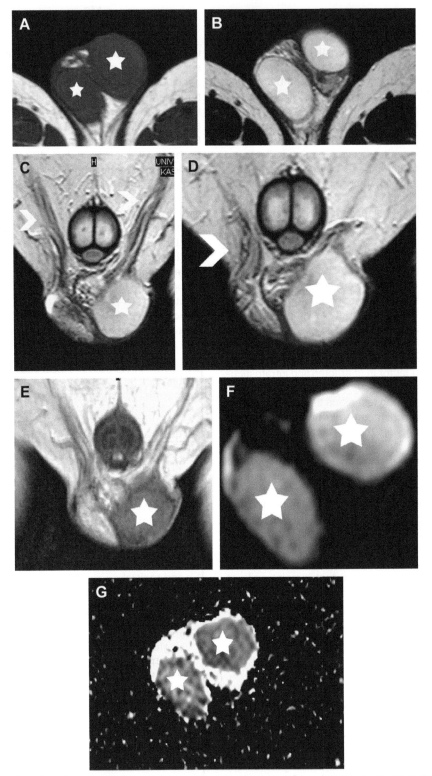

Fig. 2. Normal MR imaging examination of the scrotum in a 36-year-old man. (*A*) Transverse T1-weighted image shows normal testes (*asterisks*), with signal intensity similar to that of the surrounding muscles. (*B*) Transverse T2-weighted image. Normal testicular parenchyma (*asterisks*) appears hyperintense. The testes are surrounded by a thin hypointense halo, corresponding to tunica albuginea. (*C, D*) Coronal T2-weighted images show normal appearance of both spermatic cords (*arrowheads*). Normal left testis (*asterisk*). (*E*) Coronal DCE image depicts homogeneous enhancement of normal testicular parenchyma (*asterisk*). (*F*) Transverse DW image (*b* = 900 s/mm^2) depicts normal testes (*asterisks*) with high signal intensity. (*G*) The ADC values of normal testes (*asterisks*) are 1.04×10^{-3} mm^2/s (right testis) and 1.01×10^{-3} mm^2/s (left testis).

used for the study of human testes.[75–80] Firat and colleagues[75] showed differences in ¹H-MRS characteristics between prepubertal and postpubertal male volunteers. An increase of choline peak and a significant decrease of the lipid peak have been reported after puberty, both related to the initiation of spermatogenesis.[75] Aaronson and colleagues[76] showed a significantly high phosphocholine concentration in testes with spermatogenesis, concluding that ¹H-MRS may provide a noninvasive imaging tool in the investigation of male infertility.

NORMAL ANATOMY

Normal testes appear homogeneous, with signal intensity similar to that of the surrounding muscle on T1-weighted images (**Fig. 2**). The internal structure of testicular parenchyma is better appreciated on T2-weighted images. Normal testes appear hyperintense on T2-weighted sequences, although the signal intensity is less than that of fluid (see **Fig. 2**; **Fig. 3**). Thin radiating hypointense septa are often seen through parenchyma toward

the mediastinum testis, which is depicted as a low-signal-intensity band in the posterior aspect of the testis. The tunica albuginea appears as a thin hypointense halo surrounding the testis. Normal testis enhances moderately and homogeneously after gadolinium administration (see **Fig. 2E**), with a gradual increase of signal intensity throughout the examination (type I curve).[62–64] This behavior is probably related to an intact blood-testis barrier.[62–64] Testicular parenchyma has been reported hyperintense and slightly hypointense on high b value DWI and ADC maps, respectively, because of the complexity in histology of normal testicular parenchyma (see **Fig. 2F, G**).[70] Densely packed seminiferous tubules, lined by a compact fibroelastic connective tissue sheath and interstitial stroma, containing fibroblasts, blood vessels, lymphatics, and the Leydig cells within normal testis, are responsible for the restricted diffusion.[12,70] ADC values of the normal testis have been previously published (1.11 $\pm$ 0.18 $\times$ 10^{-3} mm²/s).[70]

The normal epididymis appears as isointense on T1- and hypointense on T2-weighted sequences,

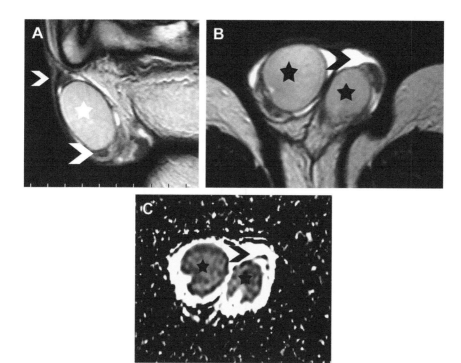

Fig. 3. Normal findings in a 21-year-old man. (*A*) Sagittal and (*B*) transverse T2-weighted images show normal hyperintensity of both testes (*asterisks*). The left epididymis (head and tail, *arrowhead*) appears hypointense. A small amount of hydrocele is noted bilaterally. (*C*) Transverse ADC map (b = 900 s/mm²) depicts hyperintensity of the left epididymal head (*arrowhead*). The ADC values of testicular parenchyma (*asterisks*) are 0.87 $\times$ 10^{-3} mm²/s (right testis) and 0.92 $\times$ 10^{-3} mm²/s (left testis), and the ADC value of the left epididymis is 1.69 $\times$ 10^{-3} mm²/s (*arrowhead*).

respectively, and is better appreciated on sagittal T2-weighted images (see **Fig. 3**). It appears with low signal intensity on DWI, and the mean ADC is $1.39 \pm 0.14 \times 10^{-3}$ mm^2/s (see **Fig. 3**C). A small hydrocele is often seen in the scrotum and is considered a physiologic finding. The spermatic cords are better evaluated on coronal T2-weighted sequences, as hyperintense structures, because of the presence of fat, with hypointense vessels coursing through them (see **Fig. 2**C, D).

Box 1
Histologic classification of malignant testicular tumors

GCTs

  Intratubular germ cell neoplasia, unclassified

  Malignant pure GCT (showing a single cell type)

    Seminoma

    Embryonal carcinoma

    Teratoma

    Choriocarcinoma

    Yolk sac tumor

  Malignant mixed GCT (showing more than one histologic type)

    Embryonal carcinoma and teratoma with or without seminoma

    Embryonal carcinoma and yolk sac tumor with or without seminoma

    Embryonal carcinoma and seminoma

    Yolk sac tumor and teratoma with or without seminoma

    Choriocarcinoma and any other element

  Polyembryoma

Sex cord and stromal tumors

  Leydig cell tumor

  Sertoli cell tumor

  Granulosa cell tumor

  Fibroma-thecoma

Tumors with both sex cord and stromal cells and germ cells

  Gonadoblastoma

Lymphoid and hematopoietic tumors

  Lymphoma

  Leukemia

Metastases

PATHOLOGY
Intratesticular Masses

Testicular tumors

Testicular carcinoma, although representing 1.0% to 1.5% of all malignancies in men, is the most common neoplasm in boys and young adults aged 15 to 34 years old.[12,87–91] The estimated number of new cases of testicular cancer in the United States during 2013 is 7920, and deaths related to testicular cancer are estimated to occur in 370 patients.[87] Testicular cancer more often presents as a painless scrotal mass.

Testicular tumors may be subdivided into GCTs and non-GCTs (**Box 1**). Most (95%) testicular carcinomas are GCTs, arising from the germinal epithelium of the seminiferous tubules.[88–91] The GCTs are fairly evenly split between seminomas and nonseminomatous GCTs (NSGCTs). Less than 50% of malignant GCTs have a single cell type, of which roughly 50% are seminomas, seen more often during the fourth decade of life. The remaining testicular tumors have more than 1 cell

---

Table 2
Staging classification of testicular cancer and assessment of primary tumor

Stage of Primary Tumor	Extent of Primary Tumor Assessed After Radical Orchiectomy
pTx	Primary tumor cannot be assessed
pT0	No evidence of primary tumor in the testis
pTis	Intratubular germ cell neoplasia or carcinoma in situ
pT1	Tumor confined to the testis, without vascular or lymphatic invasion, with or without involvement of the epididymis or rete testis: may invade the tunica albuginea but not the tunica vaginalis
pT2	Tumor confined to the testis, with or without involvement of the epididymis or rete testis, with vascular or lymphatic invasion or extension through the tunica albuginea with invasion of the tunica vaginalis
pT3	Tumor invades the spermatic cord with or without vascular or lymphatic invasion
pT4	Tumor invades the scrotal wall with or without vascular or lymphatic invasion

type.[88–91] NSGCTs include a large group of histologically diverse neoplasms, with 4 basic types, including embryonal carcinoma, teratoma, choriocarcinoma, and yolk sac tumor. NSGCTs typically occur earlier in life, usually during the third decade.[88–91]

The local extent (T) of testicular tumors is classified according to the recommendations of the European GCC Consensus Group (EGCCCG)

and is presented in **Table 2**.[58] More than 70% of GCTs are diagnosed at an early stage.

Most non–germ cell neoplasms of the testis are derived from the cells forming the sex cords (Sertoli cells) and the interstitial stroma (Leydig cells).[1,12,88–92] These neoplasms compose approximately 4% of all testicular malignancies in adults, with a higher incidence in children (10%–30%). Although they are usually benign

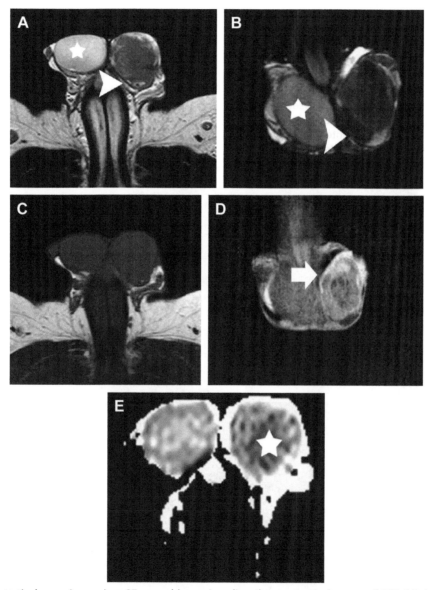

Fig. 4. Left testicular seminoma in a 27-year-old man invading the paratesticular space (pT2). (A) Axial and (B) coronal T2-weighted images show left intratesticular tumor extending into the paratesticular space (*arrowhead*). The mass is mainly homogeneous and hypointense when compared with the normal contralateral testis (*asterisk*). (C) Axial T1-weighted image fails to demonstrate the neoplasm. (D) Coronal DCE image depicts inhomogeneous tumor enhancement (*arrow*). (E) Transverse ADC map ($b = 900$ s/mm^{-2}) shows restricted tumor diffusion (*asterisk*). The ADC values of the neoplasm are 0.50×10^{-3} mm^2/s^{-1}, less than that of the normal contralateral testis (0.98×10^{-3} mm^2/s^{-1}).

(90%), the preoperative diagnosis of their nature is usually difficult.

Testicular lymphoma constitutes 1% to 9% of all testicular carcinomas but represents the most common testicular tumor in men older than 60 years. Secondary involvement of the testis in patients with an established lymphoma is much more common than primary testicular lymphoma. It is the most common bilateral testicular neoplasm, often locally invasive, typically infiltrating the epididymis, the spermatic cord, and the scrotal skin.[12,93–95] Leukemia may appear as an infiltrative epididymal-testicular mass, more often in patients with a known history of treated leukemia.[12]

MR imaging findings
Conventional MR imaging criteria used to characterize testicular malignancies include the presence of a predominantly hypointense intratesticular mass lesion on T2-weighted images when compared with the normal testis (**Fig. 4**) or a heterogeneous mass with variable signal intensity on T2-weighted images (**Fig. 5**), inhomogeneously enhancing after gadolinium administration (see **Figs. 4** and **5**).[12–18] All testicular neoplasms usually have similar signal intensity with the normal contralateral testis on T1-weighted sequences (see **Fig. 4**C). The coexistence of areas of hemorrhage and/or necrosis within the tumor (see **Fig. 5**; **Fig. 6**) as well as the extension of the neoplasm to the testicular tunicae (**Fig. 7**), the paratesticular space (see **Fig. 4**), and/or the spermatic cord (**Fig. 8**) are considered as secondary findings used to confirm the diagnosis of malignancy.[12–18]

Imaging features of testicular carcinomas closely correlate with gross morphology and histologic characteristics.[1,12,18,34] On pathology, classic seminomas are often homogeneously solid, lobulated masses, composed of uniform tumor cells with abundant clear cytoplasm. These cells are arranged in nests outlined by fibrous

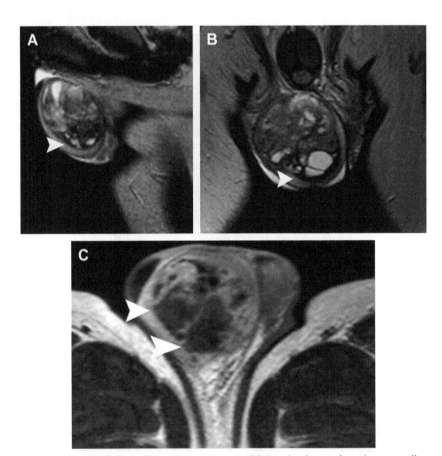

Fig. 5. Mixed germ cell tumor of the right testis in a 41-year-old man (embryonal carcinoma, yolk sac tumor, and teratoma). (*A*) Sagittal and (*B*) coronal T2-weighted images show extremely heterogeneous right intratesticular mass. The neoplasm is surrounded by a thin hypointense halo (*arrowhead*), corresponding to fibrous pseudocapsule on pathology. (*C*) Transverse contrast-enhanced T1-weighted image shows inhomogeneous tumor enhancement. Nonenhancing areas corresponded to areas of necrosis on histology (*arrowheads*).

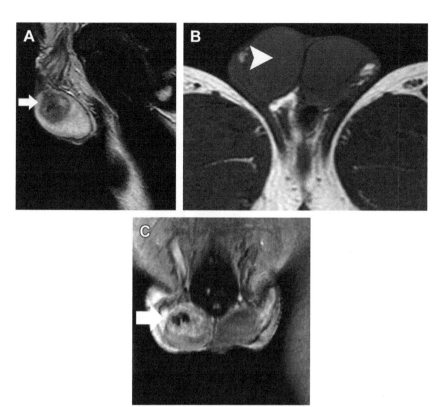

Fig. 6. Embryonal carcinoma confined to the right testis (pT1) in a 26-year-old man. (*A*) Sagittal T2-weighted image shows heterogeneous intratesticular tumor (*arrow*) surrounded by a rim of normal testicular parenchyma. (*B*) Axial T1-weighted image depicts small hyperintense area within the mass (*arrowhead*), corresponding to area of hemorrhage. (*C*) Coronal DCE image shows strong, heterogeneous tumor enhancement (*arrow*). Imaging findings are suggestive of nonseminomatous tumor.

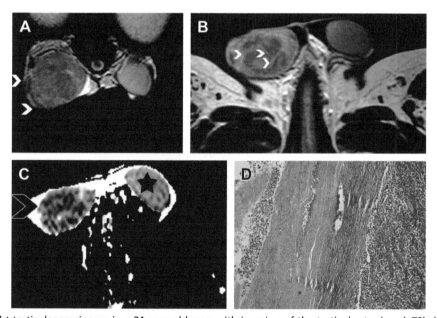

Fig. 7. Right testicular seminoma in a 31-year-old man with invasion of the testicular tunicae (pT2). (*A*) Coronal T2-weighted image depicts large right testicular tumor, invading the testicular tunicae and extending to the paratesticular space (*arrowheads*). The neoplasm is homogeneous and hypointense. (*B*) Axial postcontrast T1-weighted image shows tumor septa (*arrowheads*) enhancing more than the remaining tissue. Imaging findings are suggestive of a seminomatous lesion. (*C*) Transverse ADC map ($b = 900$ s/mm^{-2}) shows tumor hypointensity (*arrowhead*). The ADC values of testicular seminoma are 0.52×10^{-3} mm^2/s^{-1}. The ADC values of the normal contralateral testis (*asterisk*) are 0.85×10^{-3} mm^2/s^{-1}. (*D*) Histologic section (hematoxylin-eosin, original magnification $\times$ 100). Seminoma of the testis: the tumor cells infiltrate the capsule.

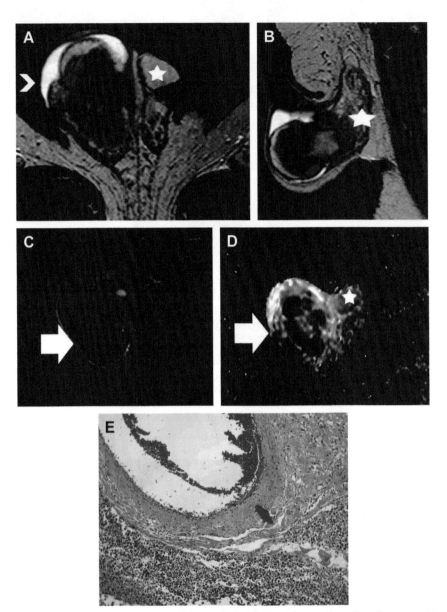

Fig. 8. Right testicular seminoma in a 41-year-old man with Down syndrome, invading the spermatic cord (pT3). (*A*) Transverse and (*B*) sagittal T2-weighted image reveals a large, heterogeneous, mainly hypointense right intratesticular mass, extending into the proximal part of the spermatic cord (*asterisk*, *B*). Small right hydrocele (*arrowhead*). Atrophic left testis (*asterisk*, *A*). (*C*) Coronal DCE image at an early phase (180 seconds) shows strong, inhomogeneous tumor enhancement (*arrow*). (*D*) Transverse ADC map ($b = 900$ s/mm^{-2}) shows tumor hypointensity (*arrow*). The ADC values of testicular carcinoma are 0.65×10^{-3} mm^2/s^{-1}. The ADC values of the contralateral testis (*asterisk*) are 1.42×10^{-3} mm^2/s^{-1}. (*E*) Histologic section (hematoxylin-eosin, original magnification $\times$ 100). Seminoma of the testis: the neoplastic cells infiltrate the seminiferous duct.

bands, usually infiltrated by lymphocytes and plasma cells.[96] Therefore, on MR imaging, seminomas are often depicted as multinodular tumors of uniform signal intensity, hypointense on T2-weighted sequences. Bandlike structures of low signal intensity on T2-weighted images, enhancing more than the remaining tumor tissue after gadolinium administration, are often seen within these neoplasms, corresponding to the fibrovascular septa (**Fig. 9**).[18,34] NSGCTs have extremely diverse histologic characteristics and, therefore, are expected to appear as heterogeneous masses on MR imaging, with areas of hemorrhage and/or necrosis, showing inhomogeneous

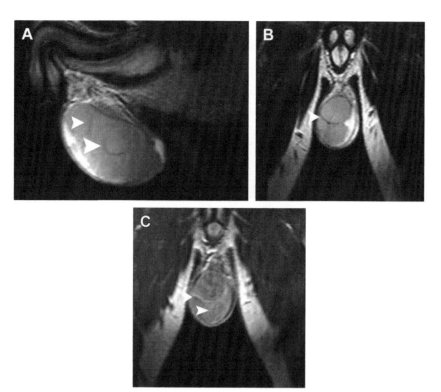

Fig. 9. Typical right testicular seminoma, confined to the testis. Sagittal (*A*) and coronal (*B*) T2-weighted images show multinodular right intratesticular mass. The tumor is mainly hypointense on T2-weighted images, with thin hypointense septa (*arrowheads*). (*C*) Coronal postcontrast T1-weighted image shows enhancement of tumor septa (*arrowheads*). Imaging findings are suggestive of seminomatous tumor.

enhancement after gadolinium administration (see **Figs. 5** and **6**). A hypointense halo on T2-weighted images may be detected at the periphery of testicular tumors, more often in NSGCTs, corresponding to a fibrous capsule on histology (see **Fig. 5**). Based on MR imaging findings, differentiation between seminomatous from nonseminomatous tumors was possible in 91% of cases in a retrospective review of 21 GCTs.[18]

On DCE MR imaging, testicular carcinomas usually show an early upstroke, followed by gradual washout of the contrast medium (type III curve, **Figs. 10** and **11**).[62–64] Testicular malignancies are often hyperintense on DW images, when compared with the usually hypointense benign scrotal lesions and even to the normally hyperintense testicular parenchyma.[70] The ADC values ($\times 10^{-3}$ mm^2/s) of intratesticular malignancies (0.85 ± 0.62) are lower than that of normal testicular parenchyma and benign intratesticular lesions (see **Figs. 4E, 7C,** and **8D**).[70] Restricted diffusion in testicular malignancies is mainly related to high tumor cellularity, densely packed neoplastic cells, and enlargement of the nuclei, all resulting in reduced mobility of water molecules.[70]

MR imaging has been reported useful in the preoperative evaluation of the local stage T in testicular carcinomas, which is particularly recommended in cases of planned TSS. The preoperative knowledge of the exact tumor dimensions, possible invasion of the rete testis or the paratesticular space and the presence of a pseudocapsule facilitating possible tumor enucleation are extremely important. According to a retrospective study of 28 testicular tumors, the local extension of testicular carcinomas evaluated by MR imaging was in agreement with the histopathologic findings in 92.8% of cases.[17] The MR imaging criteria used to assess the local extent of testicular cancer are presented in **Table 3** and some examples are given in **Figs. 4–8**.

The preoperative characterization of sex cord and stromal testicular tumors based on imaging findings is usually difficult.[12] However, benign Sertoli cell tumors have been reported as relatively homogeneous hypointense intratesticular masses on T2-weighted sequences, homogeneously enhancing after gadolinium administration, with a very fast early contrast enhancement, followed by rapid washout of the contrast medium (type III

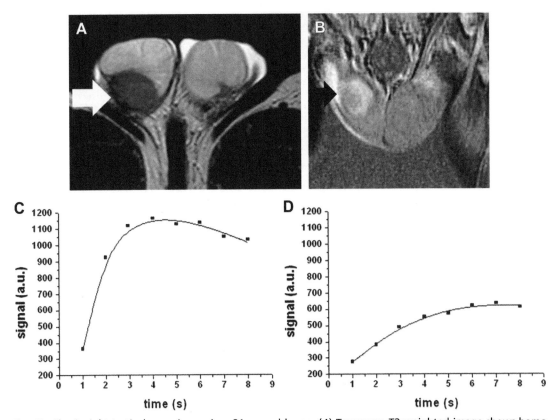

Fig. 10. Classic right testicular seminoma in a 31-year-old man. (*A*) Transverse T2-weighted image shows homogeneous, hypointense right testicular tumor (*arrow*). (*B*) Coronal DCE subtracted image at early (180 seconds) phase shows strong, heterogeneous lesion enhancement (*arrow*). (*C*) TSI plot of the neoplasm depicts avid, early contrast enhancement, followed by gradual de-enhancement (type III). (*D*) TSI plot of the normal contralateral testis (type I).

curve).[62,64,70] Diffusion imaging is useful in the differential diagnosis between Sertoli cell tumors and GCTs. Sertoli cell tumors present less restricted diffusion than GCTs.

Imaging findings of lymphomatous or leukemic infiltration of testicular parenchyma is usually nonspecific. However, the diagnosis of primary testicular lymphoma may be suggested in the presence of a hypointense intratesticular mass on T2-weighted sequences, strongly and heterogeneously enhancing after gadolinium administration, and detected in a men older than 60 years (**Fig. 12**).[94]

Benign Intratesticular Masses

Although rare, benign intratesticular mass lesions, including tubular ectasia of rete testis (TERT), epidermoid cyst, testicular infarction, fibrosis, hematoma, testicular hemorrhagic necrosis, and orchitis, should be accurately characterized to avoid unnecessary radical orchiectomy. MR imaging of the scrotum provides satisfactory results in

the differential diagnosis between benign and malignant intratesticular masses.[12,15–17] Serra and colleagues[16] reported an overall accuracy of 91% in the characterization of intratesticular lesions after inconclusive clinical and sonographic findings. In the researchers' report, MR imaging shows a high sensitivity (100%), specificity (87.5%), and accuracy (96.4%) in differentiating intratesticular masses.[17] Absence of contrast enhancement proved to be the most sensitive sign for predicting the benign nature of intratesticular masses (**Figs. 13–16**).[17] However, benign intratesticular lesions may enhance. In these cases, DCE MR imaging or DW sequences may add valuable information in the differential diagnosis.[62] Benign intratesticular masses usually exhibit strong enhancement, with a late peak, followed by either a plateau or a gradual increase of signal intensity in the delayed phase on DCE MR imaging (type II curve, **Fig. 17**).[62] No restricted diffusion and a mean ADC value ($\times 10^{-3}$ mm^2/s) of 1.56 ± 0.85 have been reported for benign intratesticular mass lesions (**Fig. 18**).[70]

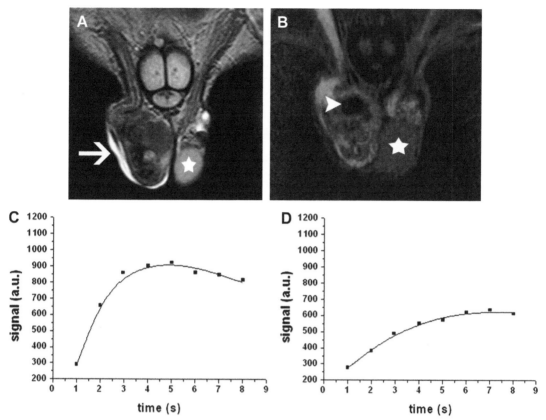

Fig. 11. Mixed germ cell tumor (embryonal carcinoma, seminoma, yolk sac tumor, and teratoma) of the right testis in a 27-year-old man. (*A*) Coronal T2-weighted image depicts heterogeneous right testicular mass, replacing the testis. Small right hydrocele (*arrow*). The contralateral normal testis (*asterisk*) enhances moderately and homogeneously. (*B*) Coronal DCE subtracted image at late (360 seconds) phase shows heterogeneous tumor enhancement, with an area of necrosis (*arrowhead*). (*C*) TSI curve of the neoplasm is suggestive of malignancy (type III). (*D*) TSI curve of the normal contralateral testis (type I).

Table 3 MR imaging criteria for local stage T of testicular cancer	
Stage of Primary Tumor	**Extent of Primary Tumor Assessed on MR Imaging**
pT1	Intratesticular tumor surrounded by a rim of normal testicular parenchyma and/or intact testicular tunicae, detected as a continuous hypointense halo in the periphery of the testis
pT2	Intratesticular tumor invading the testicular tunicae, with or without presence of mass in the paratesticular space
pT3	Enlargement and contrast-enhancement of the spermatic cord because of tumor extension
pT4	Invasion of the scrotal wall by tumor

TERT is a relatively common benign condition, which may mimic neoplasia, both clinically and sonographically.[12,17,55,56] The MR imaging findings are typical, including multicystic masses of variable size, with signal intensity similar to that of water, free diffusion, and lack of contrast enhancement (see **Fig. 13**). TERT is typically located in the mediastinum testis and it is often bilateral.[55,56]

Epidermoid cysts account for approximately 1% of all testicular masses.[12] Pathologically, it is composed of concentric layers of laminated keratinous material, which produce a characteristic target appearance on imaging. The typical MR imaging finding includes the presence of alternating zones of high and low signal intensity on T2-weighted images, corresponding to both high water and lipid content and dense keratin debris and calcifications, respectively, on pathology. Absence of contrast enhancement confirms the benignity of the lesion (see **Fig. 14**).[52–54]

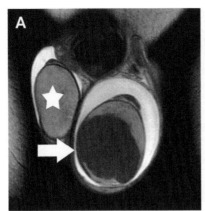
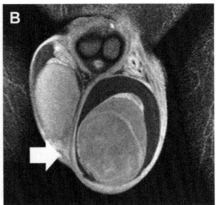

Fig. 12. Primary diffuse large B-cell testicular lymphoma in a 52-year-old man. Coronal (*A*) T2- and (*B*) contrast-enhanced T1-weighted images depict large left intratesticular mass lesion (*arrow*). The tumor is mainly hypointense on T2-weighted images, when compared with the normal contralateral testis (*asterisk, A*) and enhances heterogeneously. A moderate left hydrocele and a small right hydrocele are also noted.

Testicular fibrosis may mimic malignancy on sonographic examination. The MR imaging findings suggesting the diagnosis of testicular fibrosis are the presence of an intratesticular mass with a low on T1-weighted signal intensity and a very low T2-weighted signal intensity, not enhancing after gadolinium administration.[15–17]

Segmental testicular infarction is an infrequent testicular disease.[57] The presence of a triangular-shaped avascular intratesticular mass lesion on MR imaging, pointing toward the rete testis, hypointense on T2-weighted images, with a surrounding markedly enhancing rim may strongly suggest testicular infarction.[57] A hyperintense testis on T1-weighted images, with a very low signal intensity or with a spotty or streaked pattern of very low signal intensity on T2-weighted images and decreased or absent enhancement after contrast administration, is suggestive of hemorrhagic necrosis of the testicle (see **Fig. 15**).[17,66]

Scrotal inflammatory disease may mimic neoplasia in all phases of evolution, especially in chronic stages. It is considered the most common cause of false-positive scrotal explorations. Isolated granulomatous orchitis is a rare disease, with obscure pathogenesis.[12] Absence of contrast enhancement and restricted diffusion may be useful for considering the benign nature of this entity (see **Fig. 16**).[41]

Paratesticular Masses

MR imaging allows precise localization of scrotal masses and defines the anatomic relationship to the surrounding structures (**Fig. 19**). Most paratesticular mass lesions are benign, including cysts

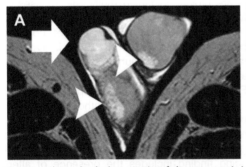
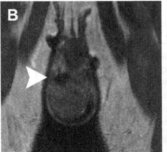
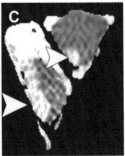

Fig. 13. Bilateral tubular ectasia of the rete testis in a 64-year-old man. (*A*) Transverse T2-weighted image shows multilocular intratesticular lesions (*arrowheads*), located in the mediastinum. The lesions have signal intensity similar to that of water. A right spermatocele (*arrow*) is also noted. Small hydrocele is seen bilaterally (physiologic finding). (*B*) Coronal DCE image depicts absence of enhancement of the right intratesticular lesion (*arrowhead*). (*C*) Transverse ADC map ($b = 900$ s/mm^{-2}). The ADC values of the normal testes are 1.30×10^{-3} mm^2/s^{-1} (*right*) and 1.32×10^{-3} mm^2/s^{-1} (*left*). Tubular ectasia of rete testis appears hyperintense on the ADC maps (*arrowheads*), with an ADC value of 2.5×10^{-3} mm^2/s^{-1} (*right*) and 2.66×10^{-3} mm^2/s^{-1} (*left*).

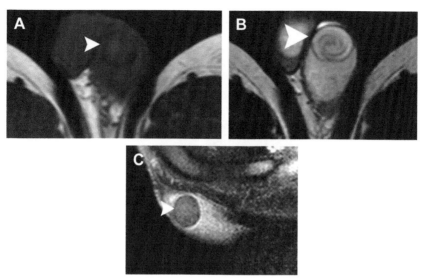

Fig. 14. Epidermoid cyst of the left testis in a 20-year-old man. (*A*) Transverse T1-weighted image shows a left intratesticular mass lesion, with smooth margins and a hyperintense area centrally (*arrowhead*), corresponding to dense keratinized material and calcifications on histology. (*B*) Transverse T2-weighted image depicts the typical onion-skin appearance of the lesion (*arrowhead*), corresponding to the laminated layers of keratinized material on pathology. Imaging findings were suggestive of an epidermoid cyst diagnosis. (*C*) Sagittal fat-suppressed T1-weighted image after gadolinium administration shows absence of lesion enhancement (*arrowhead*), a finding suggestive of benignity.

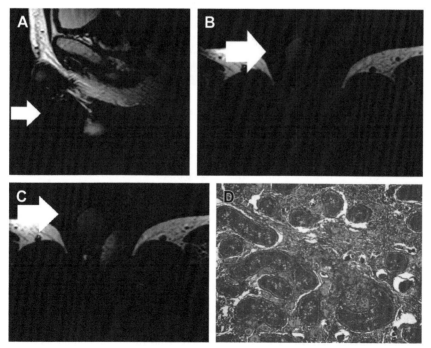

Fig. 15. Right testicular hemorrhagic necrosis in a 56-year-old man. (*A*) Sagittal T2-weighted image depicts right testis with very low signal intensity (*arrow*). (*B*) Transverse T1-weighted image demonstrates hyperintensity of right testis (*arrow*). (*C*) Transverse T1-weighted image after gadolinium administration depicts lack of enhancement of the right testis (*arrow*). (*D*) Histologic section (hematoxylin-eosin, original magnification × 100): ghost seminiferous tubules.

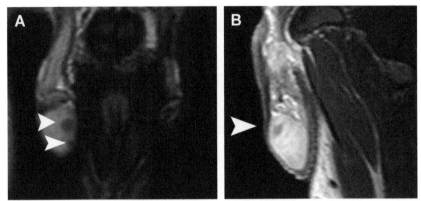

Fig. 16. Granulomatous orchitis in a 33-year-old man. (*A*) Coronal T2-weighted image depicts 2 small-sized right intratesticular mass lesions (*arrowheads*), mainly hypointense. (*B*) Sagittal postcontrast T1-weighted image shows absence of contrast enhancement (*arrowhead*), a finding suggestive of a benign diagnosis.

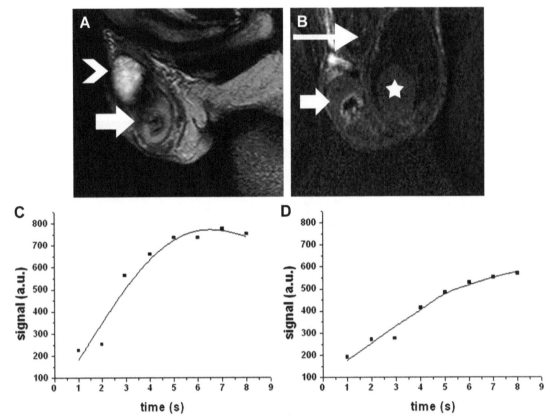

Fig. 17. Postbiopsy changes of the right testis in a 36-year-old man. Histology was negative for malignancy. (*A*) Sagittal T2-weighted image depicts heterogeneous mass lesion in the lower pole of the right testis (*arrow*). A moderate amount of hydrocele (*arrowhead*) is seen in the left hemiscrotum. (*B*) Coronal DCE subtracted image at early (180 seconds) phase demonstrates strong, heterogeneous lesion enhancement (*arrow*). Left testis (*asterisk*) enhances homogeneously. Left hydrocele (*long arrow*). (*C*) TSI curve of the intratesticular mass lesion shows an initial upstroke, followed by a plateau in the late postcontrast phase (type II). (*D*) TSI curve of the normal left testis depicts a moderate, linear increase of contrast enhancement throughout the examination (type I).

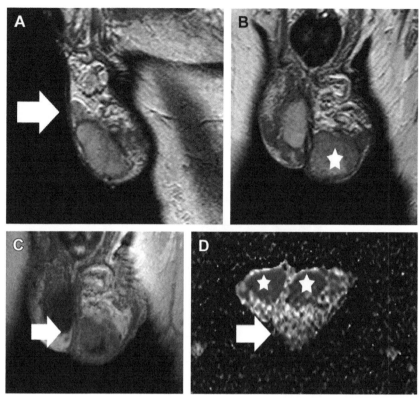

Fig. 18. Left epididymo-orchitis in a 71-year-old man. (A) Sagittal and (B) coronal T2-weighted images show enlargement and hypointensity of both the left epididymis (*arrow, A*) and the testis (*asterisk, B*). (C) Coronal DCE image depicts heterogeneous lesion enhancement (*arrow*). (D) The ADC values of the left epididymis (*arrow*) are 1.53×10^{-3} mm^2/s and that of the ipsilateral testis (*asterisk*) 0.94×10^{-3} mm^2/s, (right testis: 1.05×10^{-3} mm^2/s, *asterisk*).

and spermatoceles; scrotal fluid collections, like hydroceles and pyoceles; inflammatory lesions; and hernias.[13] In epididymitis/epididymo-orchitis, MR imaging shows a slightly high signal on T2-weighted images, increased diffusion, and inhomogeneous enhancement (see **Fig. 18**; **Fig. 20**).

Solid neoplasms of the paratesticular space are rare.[13,14,43–49,88,89] They may occur at all ages, usually presenting as slow-growing painless scrotal masses. The preoperative characterization of paratesticular tumors may be difficult. In some cases, however, MR imaging findings, in combination with tumor location, morphology, and tissue characteristics, may help to narrow the differential diagnosis. DWI may further help for lesion characterization.[70] Hypointensity on DWI and increased ADC ($1.72 \pm 0.60 \times 10^{-3}$ mm^2/s) is in favor of benign paratesticular lesions.[70]

Lipoma is the most common benign tumor of the paratesticular space, usually arising from the spermatic cord. The tumor is readily identified on MR imaging, owing to its characteristic signal intensity, high and low on T1 and fat-suppressed T1-weighted images, respectively.[13] Adenomatoid

tumor is the most common tumor of the epididymis, followed by leiomyoma.[13,48,49] Patel and Silva[49] described the MR imaging findings of an adenomatoid tumor of the tunica albuginea, appearing as a slightly hypointense mass on unenhanced T1-weighted images, enhancing after gadolinium administration.

Other rare benign paratesticular tumors include fibroma, hemangioma, neurofibroma, and papillary cystadenoma.[13] Fibrous pseudotumor is not a true neoplasm but rather a reactive proliferation of paratesticular tissue. Approximately 75% of cases arise from the tunica vaginalis and the rest from the epididymis, the spermatic cord, or the tunica albuginea. MR imaging may enable its correct characterization, as the lesion appears with low signal intensity on both T1- and T2-weighted sequences because of the fibrous tissue content.[13,43–47]

In adults, the differential diagnosis of paratesticular masses should also include malignancies, like leiomyosarcoma, fibrosarcoma, liposarcoma, and lymphoma. These neoplasms are extremely rare. Finally, metastases, most commonly from

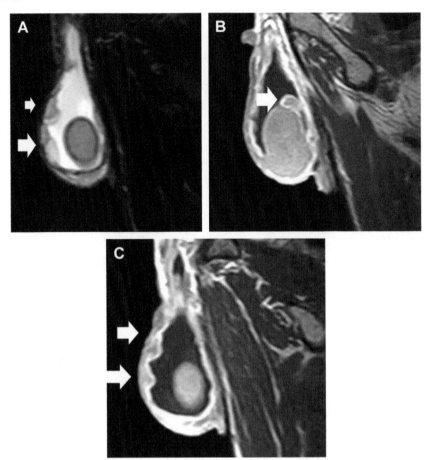

Fig. 19. Paratesticular metastases from low-grade adenocarcinoma in a 54-year-old man. Sagittal (*A*) T2 and (*B, C*) fat-suppressed postcontrast T1-weighted images show large right hydrocele and multiple nodular small-sized masses in the paratesticular space (*arrows*). The lesions have signal intensity similar to that of normal testis on T2-weighted image and enhance strongly after gadolinium administration.

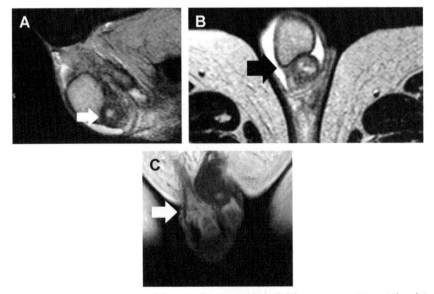

Fig. 20. Right epididymitis in a 79-year-old man. (*A*) Sagittal and (*B*) transverse T2-weighted images show enlargement and heterogeneity of the right epididymal tail (*arrow*). (*C*) Coronal DCE depicts heterogeneous enhancement of the right epididymal head (*arrow*). Imaging findings are typical of epididymitis.

testicular, prostatic, renal, and gastrointestinal primary neoplasms, should be considered, especially if there is a history of primary tumor (see **Fig. 19**).[13]

FUTURE CONSIDERATIONS/SUMMARY

Imaging of the scrotum has experienced significant advancements during the last few years. The goal is to improve the diagnosis and management of men with acute scrotal disease or a palpable mass and to reduce the number of unnecessary radical orchiectomies. Contrast-enhanced sonography has been proposed as an alternative modality in cases of inconclusive sonographic findings.[97–100] MR imaging of the scrotum, although it cannot be considered the first imaging technique in the investigation of scrotal diseases, has been proved an efficient diagnostic tool for scrotal imaging. Functional MR imaging techniques, including DCE MR imaging, DWI, and MRS, may provide additional diagnostic information in the interpretation of scrotal diseases. Large prospective studies directly comparing the diagnostic performances of sonography and MR imaging might justify the role of MR imaging in the investigation of scrotal diseases.

REFERENCES

1. Dogra VS, Gottlieb RH, Oka M, et al. Sonography of the scrotum. Radiology 2003;227(1):18–36.
2. Bhatt S, Dogra VS. Role of US in testicular and scrotal trauma. Radiographics 2008;28(6):1617–29.
3. Dogra V, Bhatt S. Acute painful scrotum. Radiol Clin North Am 2004;42(2):349–63.
4. Bhatt S, Rubens DJ, Dogra VS. Sonography of benign intrascrotal lesions. Ultrasound Q 2006;22(2):121–36.
5. Hamm B. Differential diagnosis of scrotal masses by ultrasound. Eur Radiol 1997;7(5):668–79.
6. Hamm B. Sonography of the testis and epididymis. Andrologia 1994;26(4):193–210.
7. Pavlica P, Barozzi L. Imaging of the acute scrotum. Eur Radiol 2001;11(2):220–8.
8. Tessler FN, Tublin ME, Rifkin MD. Ultrasound assessment of testicular and paratesticular masses. J Clin Ultrasound 1996;24(8):423–36.
9. Aganovic L, Cassidy F. Imaging of the scrotum. Radiol Clin North Am 2012;50(6):1145–65.
10. Cassidy FH, Ishioka KM, McMahon CJ, et al. MR imaging of scrotal tumors and pseudotumors. Radiographics 2010;30(3):665–83.
11. Mohrs OK, Thoms H, Egner T, et al. MRI of patients with suspected scrotal or testicular lesions: diagnostic value in daily practice. AJR Am J Roentgenol 2012;199(3):609–15.
12. Woodward PJ, Sohaey R, O'Donoghue MJ, et al. Tumors and tumorlike lesions of the testis: radiologic-pathologic correlation. Radiographics 2002;22(1):189–216.
13. Akbar SA, Sayyed TA, Jafri SZ, et al. Multimodality imaging of paratesticular neoplasms and their rare mimics. Radiographics 2003;23(6):1461–76.
14. Woodward PJ, Schwab CM, Sesterhenn IA. Extra-testicular scrotal masses: radiologic-pathologic correlation. Radiographics 2003;23(1):215–40.
15. Muglia V, Tucci S Jr, Elias J Jr, et al. Magnetic resonance imaging of scrotal diseases: when it makes the difference. Urology 2002;59(3):419–23.
16. Serra AD, Hricak H, Coakley FV, et al. Inconclusive clinical and ultrasound evaluation of the scrotum: impact of magnetic resonance imaging on patient management and cost. Urology 1998;51(6):1018–21.
17. Tsili AC, Argyropoulou MI, Giannakis D, et al. Magnetic resonance imaging in the characterization and local staging of testicular neoplasms. AJR Am J Roentgenol 2010;194(3):682–9.
18. Tsili AC, Tsampoulas C, Giannakopoulos X, et al. MRI in the histologic characterization of testicular neoplasms. AJR Am J Roentgenol 2007;189(6):W331–7.
19. Mattrey RF. Magnetic resonance imaging of the scrotum. Semin Ultrasound CT MR 1991;12(2):95–108.
20. Schnall M. Magnetic resonance imaging of the scrotum. Semin Roentgenol 1993;28(1):19–30.
21. Seidenwurm D, Smathers RL, Lo RK, et al. Testes and scrotum: MR imaging at 1.5 T. Radiology 1987;164(2):393–8.
22. Baker LL, Hajek PC, Burkhard TK, et al. MR imaging of the scrotum: normal anatomy. Radiology 1987;163(1):89–92.
23. Baker LL, Hajek PC, Burkhard TK, et al. MR imaging of the scrotum: pathologic conditions. Radiology 1987;163(1):93–8.
24. Rholl KS, Lee JK, Ling D, et al. MR imaging of the scrotum with a high-resolution surface coil. Radiology 1987;163(1):99–103.
25. Fritzsche PJ. MRI of the scrotum. Urol Radiol 1988;10(1):52–7.
26. Schultz-Lampel D, Bogaert G, Thüroff JW, et al. MRI for evaluation of scrotal pathology. Urol Res 1991;19(5):289–92.
27. Thurnher S, Hricak H, Carroll PR, et al. Imaging the testis: comparison between MR imaging and US. Radiology 1988;167(3):631–6.
28. Sohn M, Neuerburg J, Bohndorf K, et al. The value of magnetic resonance imaging at 1.5 T in the evaluation of the scrotal content. Urol Int 1989;44(5):284–91.
29. Sica GT, Teeger S. MR imaging of scrotal, testicular, and penile diseases. Magn Reson Imaging Clin N Am 1996;4(3):545–63.

30. Andipa E, Liberopoulos K, Asvestis C. Magnetic resonance imaging and ultrasound evaluation of penile and testicular masses. World J Urol 2004; 22(5):382–91.

31. Cramer BM, Schlegel EA, Thueroff JW. MR imaging in the differential diagnosis of scrotal and testicular disease. Radiographics 1991;11(1):9–21.

32. Müller-Leisse C, Bohndorf K, Stargardt A, et al. Gadolinium-enhanced T1-weighted versus T2-weighted imaging of scrotal disorders: is there an indication for MR imaging? J Magn Reson Imaging 1994;4(3):389–95.

33. Mäkelä E, Lahdes-Vasama T, Ryymin P, et al. Magnetic resonance imaging of acute scrotum. Scand J Surg 2011;100(3):196–201.

34. Johnson JO, Mattrey RF, Phillipson J. Differentiation of seminomatous from nonseminomatous testicular tumors with MR imaging. AJR Am J Roentgenol 1990;154(3):539–43.

35. Bhatt S, Jafri SZ, Wassermann N, et al. Imaging of non-neoplastic intratesticular masses. Diagn Interv Radiol 2011;17(1):52–63.

36. Sohaib SA, Koh DM, Husband JE. The role of imaging in the diagnosis, staging, and management of testicular cancer. AJR Am J Roentgenol 2008; 191(2):387–95.

37. Fütterer JJ, Heijmink SW, Spermon JR. Imaging the male reproductive tract: current trends and future directions. Radiol Clin North Am 2008; 46(1):133–47.

38. Fritzsche PJ, Hricak H, Kogan BA, et al. Undescended testis: value of MR imaging. Radiology 1987;164(1):169–73.

39. Kier R, McCarthy S, Rosenfield AT, et al. Nonpalpable testes in young boys: evaluation with MR imaging. Radiology 1988;169(2):429–33.

40. Miyano T, Kobayashi H, Shimomura H, et al. Magnetic resonance imaging for localizing the nonpalpable undescended testis. J Pediatr Surg 1991; 26(5):607–9.

41. Tsili AC, Argyropoulou MI, Giannakis D, et al. Isolated granulomatous orchitis: MR imaging findings. Eur J Radiol Extra 2011;79(2):e81–3.

42. Trambert MA, Mattrey RF, Levine D, et al. Subacute scrotal pain: evaluation of torsion versus epididymitis with MR imaging. Radiology 1990; 175(1):53–6.

43. Ch Tsili A, Tsampoulas C, Giannakopoulos X, et al. Solitary fibrous tumor of the epididymis: MRI features. Br J Radiol 2005;78(930):565–8.

44. Grebenc ML, Gorman JD, Sumida FK. Fibrous pseudotumor of the tunica vaginalis testis: imaging appearance. Abdom Imaging 1995;20(4): 379–80.

45. Saginoya T, Yamaguchi K, Toda T, et al. Fibrous pseudotumor of the scrotum: MR imaging findings. AJR Am J Roentgenol 1996;167(1):285–6.

46. Krainik A, Sarrazin JL, Camparo P, et al. Fibrous pseudotumor of the epididymis: imaging and pathologic correlation. Eur Radiol 2000;10(10): 1636–8.

47. Tobias-machado M, Corrêa Lopes Neto A, Heloisa Simardi L, et al. Fibrous pseudotumor of tunica vaginalis and epididymis. Urology 2000;56(4): 670–2.

48. Tsili AC, Argyropoulou MI, Giannakis D, et al. Conventional and diffusion-weighted magnetic resonance imaging findings of benign fibromatous paratesticular tumor: a case report. J Med Case Rep 2011;3(5):169.

49. Patel MD, Silva AC. MRI of an adenomatoid tumor of the tunica albuginea. AJR Am J Roentgenol 2004;182(2):415–7.

50. Tsili AC, Tsampoulas C, Giannakis D, et al. Tuberculous epididymo-orchitis: MRI findings. Br J Radiol 2008;81(966):e166–9.

51. Baker LL, Hajek PC, Burkhard TK, et al. Polyorchidism: evaluation by MR. AJR Am J Roentgenol 1987; 148(2):305–6.

52. Loya AG, Said JW, Grant EG. Epidermoid cyst of the testis: radiologic-pathologic correlation. Radiographics 2004;24(Suppl 1):S243–6.

53. Cho JH, Chang JC, Park BH, et al. Sonographic and MR imaging findings of testicular epidermoid cysts. AJR Am J Roentgenol 2002;178(3):743–8.

54. Langer JE, Ramchandani P, Siegelman ES, et al. Epidermoid cysts of the testicle: sonographic and MR imaging features. AJR Am J Roentgenol 1999;173(5):1295–9.

55. Rouviere O, Bouvier R, Pangaud C, et al. Tubular ectasia of the rete testis: a potential pitfall in scrotal imaging. Eur Radiol 1999;9(9):1862–8.

56. Tartar VM, Trambert MA, Balsara ZN, et al. Tubular ectasia of the testicle: sonographic and MR imaging appearance. AJR Am J Roentgenol 1993; 160(3):539–42.

57. Fernández-Pérez GC, Tardáguila FM, Velasco M. Radiologic findings of segmental testicular infarction. AJR Am J Roentgenol 2005;184(5):1587–93.

58. Albers P, Albrecht W, Algaba F, et al. European Association of Urology. Guidelines on testicular cancer. Updates 2011. Available at: http://www.uroweb.org/gls/pdf/11_Testicular_Cancer_LR.pdf. Accessed July 20, 2013.

59. Krege S, Beyer J, Souchon R, et al. European consensus conference on diagnosis and treatment of germ cell cancer: a report of the second meeting of the European Germ Cell Cancer Consensus Group (EGCCCG): part I. Eur Urol 2008;53(3): 478–96.

60. Krege S, Beyer J, Souchon R, et al. European consensus conference on diagnosis and treatment of germ cell cancer: a report of the second meeting of the European Germ Cell Cancer Consensus

Group (EGCCCG): part II. Eur Urol 2008;53(3): 497–513.

61. Giannarini G, Dieckmann KP, Albers P, et al. Organ-sparing surgery for adult testicular tumours: a systematic review of the literature. Eur Urol 2010; 57(5):780–90.

62. Tsili AC, Argyropoulou MI, Astrakas LG, et al. Dynamic contrast-enhanced subtraction MRI for characterizing intratesticular mass lesions. AJR Am J Roentgenol 2013;200(3):578–85.

63. Watanabe Y, Dohke M, Ohkubo K, et al. Scrotal disorders: evaluation of testicular enhancement patterns at dynamic contrast-enhanced subtraction MR imaging. Radiology 2000;217(1): 219–27.

64. Reinges MH, Kaiser WA, Miersch WD, et al. Dynamic MRI of benign and malignant testicular lesions: preliminary observations. Eur Radiol 1995; 5(6):615–22.

65. Reinges MH, Kaiser WA, Miersch WD, et al. Dynamic magnetic resonance imaging of the contralateral testis in patients with malignant tumor of the testis. Urology 1994;44(4):540–7.

66. Watanabe Y, Nagayama M, Okumura A, et al. MR imaging of testicular torsion: features of testicular hemorrhagic necrosis and clinical outcomes. J Magn Reson Imaging 2007;26(1):100–8.

67. Terai A, Yoshimura K, Ichioka K, et al. Dynamic contrast-enhanced subtraction magnetic resonance imaging in diagnostics of testicular torsion. Urology 2006;67(6):1278–82.

68. Costabile RA, Choyke PL, Frank JA, et al. Dynamic enhanced magnetic resonance imaging of testicular perfusion in the rat. J Urol 1993;149(5):1195–7.

69. Choyke PL. Dynamic contrast-enhanced MR imaging of the scrotum: reality check. Radiology 2000; 217(1):14–5.

70. Tsili AC, Argyropoulou MI, Giannakis D, et al. Diffusion-weighted MR imaging of normal and abnormal scrotum: preliminary results. Asian J Androl 2012; 14(4):649–54.

71. Kantarci M, Doganay S, Yalcin A, et al. Diagnostic performance of diffusion-weighted MRI in the detection of nonpalpable undescended testes: comparison with conventional MRI and surgical findings. AJR Am J Roentgenol 2010;195(4): W268–73.

72. Kato T, Kojima Y, Shibata Y, et al. Usefulness of MR fat-suppressed T2-weighted and diffusion-weighted imaging for the diagnosis of nonpalpable testes. J Urol 2008;179(4):387–8.

73. Kangasniemi M, Kaipia A, Joensuu R. Diffusion weighted magnetic resonance imaging of rat testes: a method for early detection of ischemia. J Urol 2001;166(6):2542–4.

74. Maki D, Watanabe Y, Nagayama M, et al. Diffusion-weighted magnetic resonance imaging in the detection of testicular torsion: feasibility study. J Magn Reson Imaging 2011;34(5):1137–42.

75. Firat AK, Uğraş M, Karakaş HM, et al. 1H magnetic resonance spectroscopy of the normal testis: preliminary findings. Magn Reson Imaging 2008; 26(2):215–20.

76. Aaronson DS, Iman R, Walsh TJ, et al. A novel application of 1H magnetic resonance spectroscopy: non-invasive identification of spermatogenesis in men with non-obstructive azoospermia. Hum Reprod 2010;25(4):847–52.

77. Yamaguchi M, Mitsumori F, Watanabe H, et al. In vivo localized 1H MR spectroscopy of rat testes: stimulated echo acquisition mode (STEAM) combined with short TI inversion recovery (STIR) improves the detection of metabolite signals. Magn Reson Med 2006;55(4):749–54.

78. Sasagawa I, Tateno T, Yazawa H, et al. Assessment of testicular function in experimental varicocele rats by phophorus-31 magnetic resonance spectroscopy. Urol Res 1998;26(6):407–10.

79. Kiricuta IC, Bluemm RG, Rühl J, et al. 31-P MR spectroscopy and MRI of a testicular non-Hodgkin lymphoma recurrence to monitor response to irradiation. A case report. Strahlenther Onkol 1994;170(6):359–64.

80. Thomsen C, Jensen KE, Giwercman A, et al. Magnetic resonance: in vivo tissue characterization of the testes in patients with carcinoma-in-situ of the testis and healthy subjects. Int J Androl 1987; 10(1):191–8.

81. Paldino MJ, Barboriak DP. Fundamentals of quantitative dynamic contrast-enhanced MR imaging. Magn Reson Imaging Clin N Am 2009; 17(2):277–89.

82. Moon M, Cornfeld D, Weinreb J. Dynamic contrast-enhanced breast MR imaging. Magn Reson Imaging Clin N Am 2009;17(2):351–62.

83. Do RK, Rusinek H, Taouli B. Dynamic contrast-enhanced MR imaging of the liver: current status and future directions. Magn Reson Imaging Clin N Am 2009;17(2):339–49.

84. Schaefer PW, Copen WA, Lev MH, et al. Diffusion-weighted imaging in acute stroke. Magn Reson Imaging Clin N Am 2006;14(2):141–68.

85. de Carvalho Rangel C, Hygino Cruz LC Jr, Takayassu TC, et al. Diffusion MR imaging in central nervous system. Magn Reson Imaging Clin N Am 2011;19(1):23–53.

86. Kim S, Naik M, Sigmund E, et al. Diffusion-weighted MR imaging of the kidneys and the urinary tract. Magn Reson Imaging Clin N Am 2008; 16(4):585–96.

87. American Cancer Society. Cancer facts and figures 2013. Available at: www.cancer.org/acs/groups/content/@epidemiologysurveillance/documents/document/acspc-036845.pdf. Accessed July 20, 2013.

88. Ulbright TM, Amin MB, Young RH. Tumors of the testis, adnexa, spermatic cord and scrotum. In: Rosai J, Sobin LH, editors. Atlas of tumor pathology, fasc 25, ser 3. Washington, DC: Armed Forces Institute of Pathology; 1999. p. 1–290.

89. Ulbright TM, Berney DM. Testicular and paratesticular tumors. In: Mills SE, Carter D, Greenson JK, et al, editors. Sternberg's diagnostic surgical pathology. Philadelphia: Lippincott Williams & Wilkins; 2010. p. 1944–2004.

90. Rosenberg SA. Cancer: principles and practice of oncology. 9th edition. Philadelphia: Lippincott Williams & Wilkins; 2011. p. 1280–301.

91. Woodward PJ, Heidenreich A, Looijenga LH, et al. Germ cell tumours. In: Eble JN, Sauter G, Epstein JI, et al, editors. Pathology and genetics of tumours of the urinary system and male genital organs. Lyon (France): IARC Press; 2004. p. 221–49.

92. Drevelengas A, Kalaitzoglou I, Destouni E, et al. Bilateral Sertoli cell tumor of the testis: MRI and sonographic appearance. Eur Radiol 1999;9(9): 1934.

93. Zicherman JM, Weissman D, Gribbin C, et al. Primary diffuse large B-cell lymphoma of the epididymis and testis. Radiographics 2005;25(1):243–8.

94. Tsili AC, Argyropoulou MI, Giannakis D, et al. Primary diffuse large B-cell testicular lymphoma: magnetic resonance imaging findings. Andrologia 2012;44(Suppl 1):845–7.

95. Liu KL, Chang CC, Huang KH, et al. Imaging diagnosis of testicular lymphoma. Abdom Imaging 2006;31(5):610–2.

96. Rosai J. Rosai and Ackerman's surgical pathology, vol. 1. 10th edition. Philadelphia: Elsevier; 2011. p. 1334–74.

97. Lock G, Schmidt C, Helmich F, et al. Early experience with contrast-enhanced ultrasound in the diagnosis of testicular masses: a feasibility study. Urology 2011;77(5):1049–53.

98. Lung PF, Jaffer OS, Sellars ME, et al. Contrast-enhanced ultrasound in the evaluation of focal testicular complications secondary to epididymitis. AJR Am J Roentgenol 2012;199(3):W345–54.

99. Valentino M, Bertolotto M, Derchi L, et al. Role of contrast enhanced ultrasound in acute scrotal diseases. Eur Radiol 2011;21(9):1831–40.

100. Bertolotto M, Derchi LE, Sidhu PS, et al. Acute segmental testicular infarction at contrast-enhanced ultrasound: early features and changes during follow-up. AJR Am J Roentgenol 2011; 196(4):834–41.

Male Pelvic MR Angiography

Patrick D. Sutphin, MD, PhD, Sanjeeva P. Kalva, MD*

KEYWORDS

- MR angiography • Male pelvis • Gadofosveset • May-Thurner • Testicular varicocele • Priapism
- USPIO • Nanoparticles

KEY POINTS

- Magnetic resonance (MR) angiography is a powerful tool in evaluating anatomy and pathology when applied to the male pelvis. MR angiography produces high-quality images of the arterial system approaching the resolution of CT angiography, without ionizing radiation.
- Additional advantages include the ability to obtain angiographic images in the absence of contrast material with non–contrast-enhanced MR angiographic techniques, which may be necessary in patients with renal disease or with allergy.
- The recent introduction of blood pool contrast agents, such as gadofosveset, has significantly improved the quality of imaging of the venous system, because it is no longer dependent on the first-pass imaging. Steady state imaging with blood pool contrast agents allows for the acquisition of superior-quality high-resolution images and other time-intensive techniques.
- The extended imaging time also allows for the testing for functional consequences of provocative maneuvers.

INTRODUCTION

The male pelvis is complex anatomically and contains many structures unique to the male anatomy, including the penis, scrotum, testicles, seminal vesicles, and prostate gland, as well as structures present in all humans, such as the bladder and rectum. These structures are dependent on a complex network of blood vessels to both supply the organs with blood and return the blood to the circulatory system. Perturbations of the vascular network can lead to diminished function of the male pelvic organs, including erectile dysfunction and diminished fertility. In extreme cases, disruption of blood flow can lead to catastrophic consequences, such as tissue loss and necrosis, as in testicular torsion or ischemic priapism. Examination of the male pelvic vasculature thus may provide valuable insight into male pelvic pathology as well as help with surgical or endovascular treatment planning. This article explores the use of MR angiography in the examination of the male pelvis.

MR angiography is a noninvasive technique, much like CT angiography, that can provide detailed characterization of the male pelvic vasculature. The main advantage of MR angiography is the lack of ionizing radiation, which means it can be performed in younger patients and repeated examinations can be done without concern for the deleterious consequences associated with ionizing radiation. Several additional advantages include the ability to perform noncontrast imaging, which can provide information on velocity and direction of blood flow and can be performed in patients with iodinated contrast allergy and those with kidney disease. In addition, the recent introduction of blood pool contrast media allows for steady state imaging, which can be used for provocative maneuvers as well as high-resolution image acquisition.

NON–CONTRAST-ENHANCED MR ANGIOGRAPHY

Non–contrast-enhanced MR angiography, unlike conventional x-ray angiography and CT angiography, does not require intravenous contrast administration. Instead, unenhanced MR

Division of Interventional Radiology, Department of Radiology, UT Southwestern Medical Center, 5323 Harry Hines Boulevard, Dallas, TX 75390-8834, USA
* Corresponding author.
E-mail address: sanjeeva.kalva@utsouthwestern.edu

Magn Reson Imaging Clin N Am 22 (2014) 239–258
http://dx.doi.org/10.1016/j.mric.2014.01.008
1064-9689/14/$ – see front matter © 2014 Elsevier Inc. All rights reserved

angiography takes advantage of the physiologic flow of blood to construct images based on flow-induced signal variations to characterize the lumen of blood vessels. Unenhanced MR techniques create images based on 2 basic characteristics of blood flow that relate to the signal of flowing blood relative to the stationary spins of static tissue. The first is referred to as amplitude effects, where the blood flowing into a chosen slice has a different longitudinal magnetization from the stationary tissue in the given slice. The signal intensity is dependent on the duration of the blood in the slice. The other characteristic is phase effects, which refers to the changes in transverse magnetization that occur as blood flows along the magnetic field gradient compared with the stationary spins of static tissue.[1,2]

Time of Flight

Amplitude effects are the basis of time-of-flight (TOF) imaging. A given slice (2-D) or slab (3-D) is selected and the stationary tissue is saturated using gradient-echo sequences with very short repetition times reducing the signal from the stationary tissue. Flowing blood, in contrast, has not been saturated and thus has high signal relative to the saturated stationary tissue. The amplitude of the signal is related to the duration of the blood in the slice, or TOF. Thus, the signal intensity is related to the velocity of the blood flow, with higher velocity flow yielding higher signal intensity. The angle of the flow through the selected slice also contributes to signal intensity. Flow perpendicular to the slice has the shortest route through the slice leading to increased signal intensity.[1,2]

As described previously, blood flowing into the selected slice from either direction produces high signal intensity; thus, the acquired images have both arterial and venous signal. The same principle of saturation of tissue can be applied to selectively image either arterial or venous flow. Signal from inflow can be reduced through the use of presaturation bands. Presaturation bands applied upstream to the selected slice saturate arterial inflow, resulting in the selective imaging of venous blood flow. Alternatively, presaturation bands applied downstream to the selected slice nullify signal from the venous blood flow, resulting in the selective imaging of arterial flow.

TOF images can be acquired through the use of either 2-D or 3-D techniques. In the 2-D technique, a stack of sequentially acquired single slices forms the basis of the image. The advantage of the single slice technique is that it permits good saturation of the stationary tissue optimizing the inflow effect, which in turn allows for the imaging of even in slow flow vessels. This method is best for flow perpendicular to the plane, because vessels not running perpendicular or even running parallel are subjected to saturation and signal is lost.

3-D TOF acquires an entire imaging volume simultaneously, usually a slab 30- to 60-mm in thickness. The benefit of 3-D TOF is the high spatial resolution and high signal-to-noise ratio. An additional benefit is that vessels running parallel are better depicted than in the 2-D method. A drawback of 3-D acquisition is the length of time the blood remains in the saturated slab. The extended transit time in the saturated slab may result in decreased blood signal intensity from the repeated radiofrequency pulses, with slow flow at greatest risk for signal loss. This technique, therefore, requires careful selection of slab thickness to optimize for the region of interest. An additional technique, multiple overlapping thin-slab acquisition (MOTSA), was designed to have the advantages of both 2-D and 3-D TOF. MOTSA is less susceptible to the signal loss because of saturation with 3-D TOF due to the thin slabs used and retains the high spatial resolution and signal-to-noise ratio. Reduced susceptibility to signal loss due to thinner acquisition slabs comes at the cost of longer acquisition times.[1]

Phase Contrast

Phase-contrast angiography is based on phase effects to produce angiographic images. A bipolar gradient is applied in gradient-echo acquisitions. Stationary tissue is dephased and rephased to its original state, whereas moving tissue dephases in proportion to the flow velocity. Because the encoding gradients are defined to encode flows within a certain velocity range, the operator must determine the anticipated velocity to choose the appropriate encoding gradient because velocities outside of the range are poorly encoded.[1,2]

Phase-contrast acquisitions allow for the detection of flow in any plane in 3-D space. This is accomplished by repeating the encoding in the X, Y, and Z axes. The images acquired from the 3 axes are then summed and subtracted from reference images performed without encoding gradient, leaving only the images of vessels. In addition, flow velocity can be determined noninvasively with phase-contrast imaging when the slice acquisition is perpendicular to the direction of blood flow. Flow rate can then be calculated from the product of the vessel area and flow velocity.[2]

CONTRAST-ENHANCED MR ANGIOGRAPHY
Gadolinium-Based Contrast Agent

Classically, contrast-enhanced MR angiography has been performed with extracellular contrast agents, such as gadobenate dimeglumine (Multi-Hance [Bracco Diagnostics, Monroe Township, NJ, USA]) or gadopentetate dimeglumine (Magnevist [Bayer Health Care, Whippany, NJ, USA]). Extracellular contrast agents have a short blood pool half-life and rapidly distribute into the extravascular space, thus only allowing for first-pass images, making the timing of the bolus injection relative to imaging sequence exceedingly important, with little margin for error. The rapid extravasation of contrast into the extravascular space also limits the ability to obtain high-resolution images due to the length of time required for imaging.[3,4]

The limitations of imaging with extracellular agents led to the development of contrast agents with a prolonged intravascular half-life, referred to as blood pool contrast agents. Gadofosveset (Ablavar, Lantheus Medical Imaging, Inc, North Billerica, MA, USA), previously known as Vasovist and MS-325, is the first blood pool contrast agent approved for MR angiography by the Food and Drug Administration (FDA), in December 2008, and by the European Union, in 2005. Gadofosveset is a linear ionic gadolinium chelate, which reversibly binds to human serum albumin, which effectively prolongs the serum half-life by tethering the molecule in the intravascular space and protecting it from glomerular filtration.

Prior to its approval by the FDA, gadofosveset underwent extensive clinical testing. Clinical testing included dose-escalation studies, blinded placebo-controlled studies, and 4 phase III studies. Shamsi and colleagues[5] provides a review of the safety of gadofosveset in 767 patients evaluated in phase II and phase III studies. They found that the safety profile was comparable with that of other gadolinium agents. The 3 most common adverse effects reported by the patients were pruritis (5.0%), headache (4.3%), and nausea (4.2%). Four (0.5%) of 767 patients reported 5 serious adverse events. The serious adverse events reported were chest pain, gangrene, anaphylactoid reaction, and, in one patient, hypoglycemia and aggravated coronary artery disease. Gangrene and chest pain were thought unrelated to gadofosveset. The anaphylactoid reaction resulted in itching and heavy soreness in the patient's perineal region immediately after bolus injection, which resolved within 5 minutes after intravenous administration of antihistamine, and the patient continued with the MR examination.[5]

The T1 relaxivity of gadofosveset is greater than the extracellular contrast agents in routine use. For example, gadofosveset has a T1 relaxivity in blood at 1.5 T, approximately 5-fold that of gadopentetate. The relative increased T1 relaxivity compared with other agents allows for a lower dose of contrast (0.03 mmol/kg) versus the 0.1 mmol/kg for most gadolinium-based extracellular contrast agents.[3,6,7]

Like other bolus-injectable contrast media, first-pass MR angiography is easily performed with gadofosveset. The principal advantage of gadofosveset is the ability to perform steady state imaging, providing the opportunity to acquire images for approximately 45 to 60 minutes after a single bolus injection. This allows for the acquisition of time-intensive acquisitions, such as high-resolution images, cardiac-gated imaging, and imaging with provocative maneuvers.[4,8] In addition, the extended period available for imaging allows for the imaging of vasculature at multiple anatomic sites.

Ultrasmall Paramagnetic Iron Oxide Particles

An alternative to gadolinium-based blood pool contrast agents is the use of ultrasmall paramagnetic iron oxide particles (USPIOs). USPIOs were initially developed by size fractionation of superparamagnetic iron oxide particles with gel chromatography, resulting in 70% of the particles smaller than 10 nm in size.[9] The reduced particle size significantly increased the blood pool half-life as well as enabling the particles to cross the capillary endothelium into the interstitial space where particles ultimately accumulate in lymph nodes.[10] The USPIOs have been extensively studied in lymphotropic nanoparticle MR imaging as a method to characterize lymph nodes as either benign or malignant in cancer patients and have demonstrated a good safety profile.[11] The T1-shortening property of the nanoparticles along with the prolonged blood pool half-life allows for the mapping of the vasculature using T1-weighted gradient-recalled echo sequences.[12] In 2009, ferumoxytol, a third-generation bolus-injectable USPIO, was approved by the FDA for the treatment of iron-deficiency anemia in adult patients with chronic kidney disease.[13] Ferumoxytol has a 10- to 14-hour blood pool half-life and is bolus injectable, allowing for first-pass as well as equilibrium-phase MR angiography.[14] Although ferumoxytol has not been specifically approved for use in MR angiography, its safety profile in patients with renal disease suggests that in patients with chronic kidney disease ferumoxytol may be a suitable substitute for gadolinium-based contrast agents. Sigovan and colleagues[15] compared TOF MR angiography with ferumoxytol-enhanced MR angiography and found consistently superior image quality with the USPIO-based blood pool agent relative to TOF.

ARTERIAL SYSTEM
Anatomy

Understanding pelvic artery anatomy and its variations is important in the interpretation of pelvic MR angiography because the arterial anatomy may have important clinical implications as well as providing guidance in preprocedural planning either for surgery or endovascular approach. The main arterial supply to the pelvic organs and lower extremities originates at approximately the L4 level with the bifurcation of the aorta into the right and left common iliac arteries. The common iliac artery measures, on average, approximately 1.23 cm in men and 1.02 cm in women[16] and courses inferolaterally along the medial border of the psoas muscle. The common iliac artery gives rise to the external and internal iliac arteries at the pelvic brim (**Fig. 1**).

External iliac artery

The external iliac artery provides the arterial supply to the lower extremity and to the tissues of the lower abdominal wall. The course of the external iliac artery continues along the medial border of the psoas muscle and as it exits the pelvis at the inguinal ligament the artery continues as the common femoral artery providing the blood supply to the lower extremity. The deep circumflex iliac artery and the inferior epigastric artery are branches

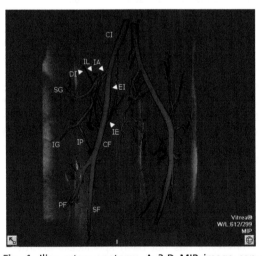

Fig. 1. Iliac artery anatomy. A 3-D MIP image constructed from first-pass MR angiography with the arteries demonstrated in red. The arterial anatomy is labeled as follows: CF, common femoral artery; CI, common iliac artery; DI, deep circumflex iliac artery; EI, external iliac artery; IA, internal iliac artery; IE, inferior epigastric artery; IG, inferior gluteal artery; IL, iliolumbar artery; IP, internal pudendal artery; PF, profunda femoral artery; SF, superficial femoral artery; SG, superior iliac artery.

of the external iliac artery that feed the muscles and skin of the lower abdomen. The deep circumflex iliac artery arises laterally from the external iliac artery and follows the course of the iliac crest of the pelvis, whereas the inferior epigastric artery branches medially just superior to the inguinal ligament and ascends superiorly in the abdominal wall (see **Fig. 1**).

Internal iliac artery

Embryologically, the internal iliac artery, sometimes still referred to as the hypogastric artery, is derived from the umbilical artery. Postnatally, after the cessation of placental circulation, the distal segment of the umbilical artery becomes the medial umbilical ligament and the proximal segment persists as the internal iliac artery and superior vesical artery.[17,18] The internal iliac artery is the predominant arterial supply to the pelvic organs and musculature of the pelvis and is subject to significant anatomic variation. Conceptually and anatomically, the branching pattern of the internal iliac artery can be divided into the anterior and posterior divisions. The posterior division supplies the musculature and osseous structures of the pelvis through the superior gluteal artery, iliolumbar artery, and lateral sacral arteries. The anterior division provides blood supply to the pelvic organs, such as the bladder and rectum, as well as the prostate, seminal vesicles, ejaculatory ducts, and penis in men (see **Fig. 1**).

Several classification schemas have been developed for the categorization of the internal iliac artery variant anatomy.[18] The Yamaki classification system described in 1998 simplifies internal iliac artery classification based on the branching patterns of the superior gluteal, inferior gluteal, and internal pudendal arteries. Yamaki initially evaluated the Adachi classification in 645 pelvic halves in Japanese cadavers and found some branching patterns different from that described in the Adachi classification system. The Yamaki classification was thus developed to simplify the classification of the internal iliac artery into 4 groups of anatomic variants. Schematic representations of the 4 groups are shown in **Fig. 2**. In group A (80% of cadaveric study), the superior gluteal artery arises independently whereas the inferior gluteal and internal pudendal arteries arise from a common trunk. Group B (15% cadaveric study) has a common posterior gluteal trunk from which the superior and inferior gluteal arteries arise with an independent origin of the internal pudendal artery. Independent origins of the superior gluteal, inferior gluteal, and internal pudendal arteries characterize group C, noted in 5.3% of the cadavers. Finally, in group D, only noted in 1

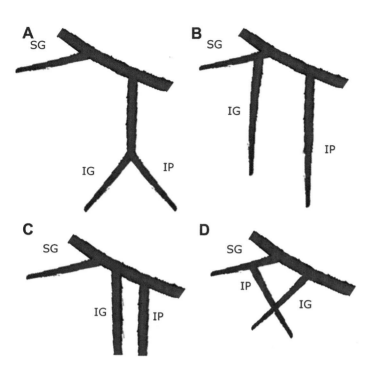

Fig. 2. Yamaki internal iliac artery classification. (*A*) The superior gluteal artery has an independent origin and the inferior gluteal artery and internal pudendal artery arise from a common trunk. (*B*) The superior and inferior gluteal arteries arise from a common trunk and the internal pudendal artery has an independent origin. (*C*) The superior gluteal, inferior gluteal and internal pudendal arteries arise independently. (*D*) The superior gluteal artery and the internal pudendal artery arise from a common trunk and the inferior gluteal artery arises independently. IG, inferior gluteal artery; IP, internal pudendal artery; SG, superior gluteal artery.

of 645 pelvic halves, the superior gluteal and internal pudendal arteries have a common origin and the inferior gluteal artery arises independently.[19–21]

The superior gluteal artery is the largest branch of the internal iliac artery and supplies the gluteal muscles—maximus, medius, and minimus. It exits the pelvis at the superior aspect of the great sacrosciatic foramen above the piriformis muscle. The second largest branch of the internal iliac artery is the inferior gluteal artery, which provides blood supply to the gluteus maximus, piriformis, and quadratus femorus muscles and exits at the inferior aspect of the greater sacrosciatic foramen inferior to the piriformis muscle. The internal pudendal artery tends to be the third largest vessel of the internal iliac artery. The course of the internal pudendal artery is similar to that of the inferior gluteal artery as it exits the inferior aspect of the great sacrosciatic foramen, but it then curves around the sacrospinous ligament and re-enters the pelvis through the lesser sacrosciatic foramen.[20] In the pelvis, the internal pudendal artery branches into the inferior rectal artery, perineal artery, and posterior scrotal branches and terminates as the common penile artery.[22]

The obturator artery is an additional branch of the internal iliac artery but is subject to considerable anatomic variation. In approximately two-thirds of cases, the obturator artery arises from the internal iliac artery and extends to and exits the obturator foramen and divides into the anterior and posterior branches in a distinctive 90° angle. In the other one-third of cases, the obturator artery is a branch of the inferior epigastric artery from the external iliac artery, a variant sometimes referred to as the *corona mortis*, translated as the crown of death due to its susceptibility to traumatic injury.[20,23,24] Additional branches of the internal iliac artery that arise from the anterior division include the superior vesical, inferior vesical, and middle rectal arteries.

Peripheral Vascular Disease

The noninvasive characterization of the patency of peripheral vasculature is an important application of MR angiography, with implications in the diagnosis of peripheral vascular disease as well as the appropriate selection of therapy. A prospective study was performed that compared both first-pass MR angiography and steady state MR angiography with gadofosveset in 334 arterial segments in 27 patients with digital subtraction angiography (DSA). First-pass MR angiography underestimated stenosis in 4.5% of the arterial segments and overestimated stenosis in 8% of the segments. High-resolution steady state imaging, however, was in agreement with DSA findings in 100% of the 334 arterial segments.[25] The improved accuracy was attributed to the high-resolution sequences that reduced volume averaging artifact only possible in steady state imaging. A maximum intensity projection (MIP) image from first-pass MR angiography is shown in comparison with a DSA image in **Fig. 3**.

Iliac Artery Aneurysms

MR angiography is useful not only for characterizing the complex vascular anatomy of the male pelvis but also for evaluating the vessels for aneurysm, dissection, stenosis, and occlusion. Isolated or solitary aneurysms of the iliac arteries have a strong male predominance with an age-related increase in incidence. Aneurysm is derived from the Greek roots, *ana* (upon) and *eurys* (broad).[26] In practical terms, aneurysm is often defined as the permanent focal dilation of the artery having at least a 1.5-times increase in diameter compared with the normal artery.[27,28] In the context of the common iliac artery, aneurysm is defined by the Society for Vascular Surgery reporting standards as any permanent focal dilation of the iliac artery greater than 1.5 cm in diameter.[26,27]

Iliac artery aneurysms are seen in approximately 10% to 20% of patients with abdominal aortic aneurysms, whereas isolated iliac artery aneurysms are rare, accounting for less than 2% of all aneurysmal disease.[29,30] Iliac artery aneurysms are important to consider and recognize due to the risk of rupture and high mortality associated with rupture. As many as 33% of patients with iliac artery aneurysms present with rupture. A majority of patients with isolated iliac artery aneurysms, however, are either asymptomatic or have nonspecific symptoms. Nonspecific symptoms are often secondary to mass effect or compressive symptoms from the aneurysm, including lumbosacral pain, tenesmus, or constipation and urinary obstruction.[28] Additional symptoms may include vascular symptoms, such as intermittent claudication, lower extremity pain from arterial occlusion, deep venous thrombosis (DVT) from iliac vein compression, or even high-output cardiac failure from arteriovenous fistula (AVF) from the erosion of the aneurysm into the iliac vein.[28] Thus, most iliac artery aneurysms are found incidentally either during surgery on diagnostic imaging studies.[30] Those patients presenting with rupture may have abrupt onset of abdominal, groin, or thigh pain and hypotensive shock.[28]

As discussed previously, there is a strong male predilection for isolated iliac artery aneurysms, with an estimated male-to-female ratio of 7:1.[26] Moreover, the incidence increases significantly with age, as evidenced by a 6.5-fold increase in incidence in patients 75 years and older compared with 55-year-old patients.[28] Thus, a typical patient with isolated iliac artery aneurysm is an elderly man in his 7th or 8th decade of life. Surveillance MR angiography from an 83-year-old man with incidentally discovered isolated right common iliac artery aneurysm is shown in **Figs. 4** and **5**. A vast majority of iliac artery aneurysms are secondary to degenerative changes resultant of atherosclerotic

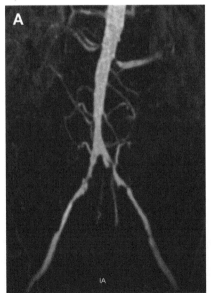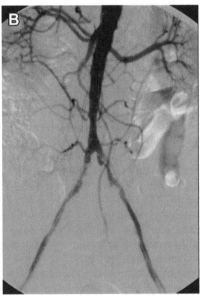

Fig. 3. Atherosclerotic disease. (*A*) MIP image from contrast-enhanced first-pass MR angiography demonstrating narrowing at the aortic bifurcation with multifocal segments of moderate to severe stenosis in the bilateral iliac arteries. (*B*) DSA prior to iliac artery stenting for comparison of findings.

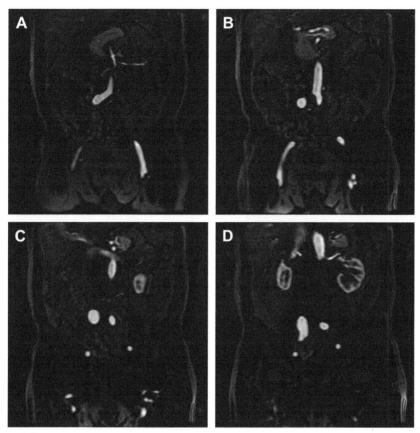

Fig. 4. Sequential fat-suppressed contrast-enhanced coronal images anterior (*A*) to posterior (*D*) demonstrate a right common iliac artery aneurysm.

disease. Additional causes include para-anastomotic graft failure, penetrating injury from trauma, and iatrogenic causes related to surgery. Other reported causes include mycotic/infectious, vasculitis, and inherited disorders of connective tissue, including Marfan syndrome and Ehler-Danlos syndrome.[26,28,29]

The expected evolution of iliac artery aneurysms is the continued expansion of the aneurysm until eventual rupture, with the risk of rupture increasing as the aneurysm progresses in size. The estimated growth rate for iliac aneurysms less than 3 cm is 1.1 mm/y and increases as the aneurysm increases in size, with estimated growth rate of 2.6 mm/y for aneurysms 3 to 5 cm in size.[26,31] The average size at time of rupture is 5.6 cm.[26] The smallest reported iliac artery aneurysm rupture was 3 cm, with none less than 3 cm reported.[29,30] Thus, the threshold for elective repair is approximately 3.5 cm or greater or when the aneurysm measures 3 to 4 cm with symptoms.[28,31] For aneurysms greater than or equal to 5 cm in size, expeditious repair is recommended to reduce the chance of rupture, especially given the high mortality associated with

emergent repair of a ruptured aneurysm estimated to be approximately 50% compared with 1% to 5% for elective repair.[30]

Endovascular repair is increasingly applied to iliac artery aneurysm repair and offers decreased hospital time, lower morbidity, and can be performed in patients with severe cardiopulmonary disease.[28] The goal of endovascular approach is to exclude the aneurysm from circulation with a stent graft. Coil embolization may also be used to prevent type II endoleak, particularly from the internal iliac artery. When interpreting pelvic MR angiography for iliac artery aneurysms, it is important to make note of several factors important for planning repair via an endovascular approach. These include the presence of an aortic aneurysm, contralateral iliac aneurysm, and involvement of the ipsilateral internal iliac artery. Additionally, careful attention to the length of normal artery proximal and distal to the aneurysm is important because at least 1.5 to 2 cm of landing zone is necessary to create a seal to prevent type I endoleak.[29,31]

Aneurysms of the external iliac artery are rare, whereas aneurysms of the common iliac artery

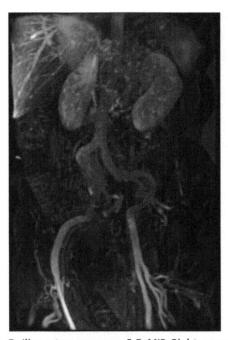

Fig. 5. Iliac artery aneurysm 3-D MIP. Right common iliac artery aneurysm. 3-D MIP image from first-pass angiography demonstrates a right common iliac artery aneurysm measuring 2.9 cm.

represent 70%, and aneurysms of the internal iliac artery represent 20% to 25% of iliac disease.[26,31] A possible explanation that has been provided is the difference in embryologic origin between the external iliac artery and the common and internal iliac arteries. The external iliac artery is derived from the iliofemoral system, whereas the common and internal iliac arteries arise from the sciatic system. During embryonic development, the internal iliac arteries provide blood supply to the pelvic organs and initially the lower extremity limb bud, but as this contribution to the lower limb degenerates the supply to the lower limb is taken over by the external iliac artery.[26,31,32]

VENOUS SYSTEM

In addition to characterization of the arterial system, MR angiography is also a useful method for the characterization and evaluation of venous system pathology. The introduction of blood pool contrast agents to MR angiography has dramatically simplified the acquisition of diagnostic-quality images of the venous system. Prior to the availability of blood pool contrast agents, the timing of injection to imaging left little margin for error in obtaining images in the optimal phase for venous enhancement. The increased half-life of contrast agents in the blood pool, such as gadofosveset, in contrast, allows for multiple acquisitions of the arterial and venous system in the steady state phase. This is advantageous in that the MR angiography can then become a functional dynamic study. For example, in patients evaluated for thoracic outlet syndrome, imaging of the subclavian vessels can be performed with arms positioned above the head and lowered in the steady state phase of contrast after a single-injection.[33] The increased time of imaging also allows for troubleshooting to optimize image quality.

The most common indication to evaluate the venous system with pelvic MR angiography at the authors' institution is to evaluate for occult DVT in patients with a negative lower extremity venous ultrasound with symptoms of lower extremity swelling, history of pulmonary embolus, or cryptogenic stroke. Additional indications include evaluation for testicular varicocele/pelvic congestions syndrome and, in a rare number of cases, priapism.

May-Thurner Syndrome

Rudolf Ludwig Karl Virchow was a mid–19th-century physician and pathologist credited with coining the terms, *thrombosis* and *embolus*. He demonstrated that masses in blood vessels were the result of thrombosis and was the first to demonstrate that the thrombus or portions thereof could detach and migrate—embolus.[34] In addition, the discrepancy in the frequency of the laterality of iliofemoral DVT, left 5 times greater than right, was explained as early as 1851 by Virchow as secondary to compression of the left iliac vein by the overlying artery.[35] In 1957, May and Thurner performed a large-scale autopsy series of 430 cadavers to more thoroughly evaluate Virchow's assumption that diminished flow on the left secondary to compression by the overlying artery is adequate to explain the predominance of left-sided iliofemoral DVT. In the autopsy series, May and Thurner identified in 22% of the cadavers a spur-like projection in the left common iliac vein at the mouth of the inferior vena cava (IVC). On microscopic examination, the spur-like projection was found composed of fibrocytes with an intermediary layer of collagen deposition, resembling a callus-like formation. The spur is now recognized as secondary to intimal hyperplasia.[36] Although this spur-like projection had been previously described by McMurrich in 1906 and 1908, the presence of this spur in the context of iliac vein thrombosis was not fully appreciated and was thought likely congenital in etiology. Based on the absence of the iliac vein spur in the 88 examined embryos and newborns and the histologic resemblance to a callus, May and Thurner concluded that the spur is an acquired defect in the course of extrauterine life.[37]

Three types of spurs were identified in the series of 430 cadavers. The first was found to protrude into the lumen of the left iliac vein like a pillar, whereas the second type of spur divides the lumen completely, and, finally, the third type of spur leads to near occlusion of the left iliac vein. The functional significance of the spur formation is narrowing of the lumen of the left common iliac vein, further hampering blood flow leading to an environment more favorable for thrombus formation.[35] The incidence of the left common iliac vein spur in the cadaver study was 22%, with no spurs identified on the right side.

May-Thurner syndrome (MTS) is most commonly asymptomatic until presentation with DVT. Additional, less-frequent presenting symptoms include left lower extremity pain, swelling, and/or symptoms of left lower extremity venous insufficiency, including varicosities and venous ulcerations.[36,38] The syndrome is usually seen in women 20 to 40 years old.[39] Raju and Neglen found a 4:1 female-to-male ratio of nonthrombotic iliac vein lesions (NIVLs) in patients with chronic venous disease.[40] Given the high prevalence of iliac vein spurs in the general population, iliac vein compression comprises only a small portion of lower extremity DVT, estimated at 2% to 3%.[39]

Pelvic MR angiography is an effective noninvasive means for evaluating for features of MTS. It should be noted that there is no widely accepted diagnostic imaging definition of MTS. MR venography features which are closely evaluated include the degree of iliac vein compression, presence of venous collaterals and direction of venous flow. Routine visualization of the spur lesion described as part of MTS is not currently possible.

The significance of iliac vein compression alone is unclear. For example, in a study of 50 consecutive patients presenting to an emergency department with abdominal pain and evaluated with CT scans, 24% of the patients had greater than 50% compression of the left common iliac vein, prompting the investigators to suggest iliac vein compression represents a normal variant.[41] Another study evaluated the degree of left iliac vein compression in 36 patients diagnosed with MTS by MRV on cross-sectional studies obtained for different reasons within 6 months of the MRV or any time after the MRV. McDermott and colleagues[42] found that the degree of left common iliac vein compression was not stable and, in fact, decreased from a mean of 62% on the MRV to 39% on the other cross-sectional studies. Thus, although the degree of iliac vein compression is a main consideration for the diagnosis of

MTS, it should be interpreted with caution in the diagnosis of MTS.

The presence of an extensive pelvic venous collateralization network diverting flow from the left common iliac vein into the lumbar veins or the veins of the pelvis is also indicative of a hemodynamically significant lesion with the presence of a mature collateral network also suggesting a chronic process.

The degree of iliac vein compression and extent of venous collateralization can be evaluated on either CT or MR imaging. A distinct advantage of MR imaging over CT is the functional analysis of flow with diagnostic sequences, such as TOF. TOF enables the evaluation of flow direction of the veins of the pelvis. In the context of MTS, the direction of flow in the left common iliac vein and left internal iliac vein are particularly important. Antegrade flow both in the left common iliac vein and left internal iliac vein suggests that the compression of the iliac vein is not hemodynamically significant. Alternatively, if there is reversal of flow, demonstrated by absence of signal, in either the left internal iliac vein or the left common iliac vein, this suggests that normal flow is hindered indicating a hemodynamically significant lesion from compression and/or spur lesion.

Additional diagnostic evaluation is generally performed immediately prior to treatment of left iliac vein compression with stenting. This can be performed with contrast-enhanced venography and intravascular ultrasound (IVUS). Venography allows for the functional assessment of the drainage pattern of the left lower extremity as well as the direction of flow and the presence of venous collateral networks. The added advantage of IVUS to the venography allows for the assessment of the degree of left common iliac vein compression and in many cases for direct visualization of the spur.[36] IVUS is also useful for planning of stent placement in choosing a stent diameter and length.[43] Endovascular treatment with stenting is currently the preferred method of treatment because it has been found in small studies to be safe and effective as well as provide relief of acute symptoms.[44,45]

A 21-year-old man with history of left lower extremity varicose veins presented with worsening bulging varicose veins over the prior 3 months and with increasing discomfort and heaviness in his left lower extremity. MR angiography revealed compression of the left common iliac vein by greater than 50% with extensive venous collateralization and reversal of flow in the left internal iliac vein (see **Fig. 6**). He was subsequently taken for venography and IVUS, which confirmed iliac vein compression with reversal of flow in the left internal iliac vein (**Fig. 7**A, B). The left common iliac vein

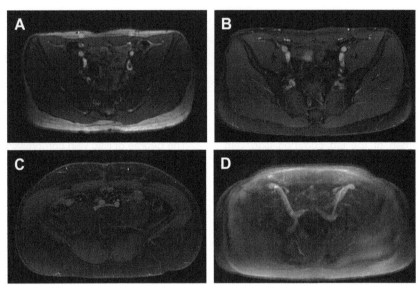

Fig. 6. MTS. (*A*) TOF image with apparent filling defect in the left common iliac vein. (*B*) Contrast-enhanced (gadofosveset) fat-suppressed image demonstrates enhancement of the common iliac vein suggesting apparent filling defect on TOF imaging is likely related to slow flow. (*C*) Fat-suppressed contrast-enhanced image with marked flattening of the common iliac vein between the right common iliac artery and the fifth vertebral body. (*D*) TOF MIP image with absence of left internal iliac vein indicating either reversal of flow or slow flow in the left internal iliac vein.

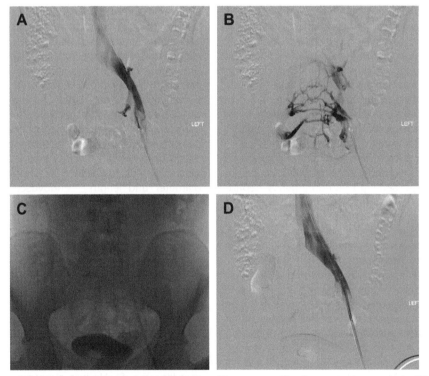

Fig. 7. Endovascular treatment of MTS. (*A*) Left common iliac venography demonstrates reversal of flow into the left internal ilia vein as well as (*B*) flow into collateral pelvic veins. (*C*) An 18-mm × 6-cm bare-metal stent was placed in the left common iliac vein. (*D*) Poststent images demonstrate antegrade flow in the left common iliac vein with resolution of flow to the pelvic collaterals.

was stented with a bare-metal stent and improved flow in the left common iliac vein was demonstrated on poststenting images (see **Fig. 7**C, D).

Right Iliac Vein Compression

Although less common than left common iliac vein compression, symptoms and DVT have also been reported to arise in the setting of right iliac vein compression. In a study of NIVLs, a nonspecific term often used to refer to both extrinsic and intrinsic lesions, Raju and Neglen performed IVUS examination in 879 chronic venous disease patients with severe symptoms. They found iliac vein obstructive lesions in 938 limbs with a ratio of left to right lesions of 3:1. The right common iliac artery crosses the left common iliac vein abruptly and sandwiches it between the L5 vertebral body posteriorly, whereas the course of the right iliac artery over the right iliac vein is more variable and tends to have a longer overlay of the right iliac vein. NIVLs may arise either proximally or distally in the right iliac vein.[40]

A 53-year-old avid male cyclist presented with worsening shortness of breath and diminished cycling capacity and was found to have bilateral pulmonary emboli. Lower extremity ultrasound demonstrated an occlusive thrombus within the right common femoral vein (**Fig. 8**A). A subsequent

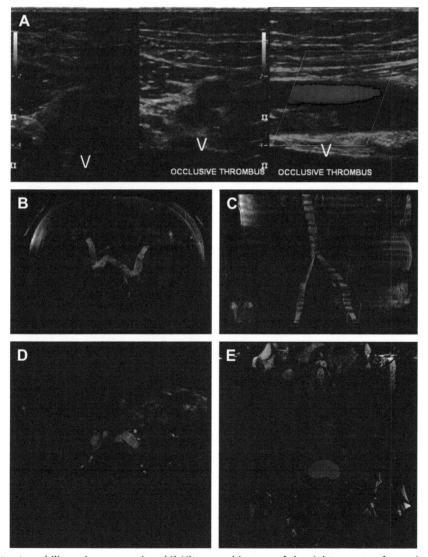

Fig. 8. Right external iliac vein compression. (*A*) Ultrasound images of the right common femoral vein demonstrate echogenic occlusive thrombus in the right common femoral vein. (*B, C*) TOF MIP images in the axial and coronal projections demonstrate the absence of the right internal iliac vein either due to reversal of flow or slow flow. (*D, E*) Fat-suppressed gadofosveset-enhanced images performed in the steady state demonstrated flattening of the right external iliac vein in the axial and coronal planes.

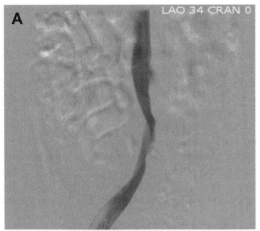

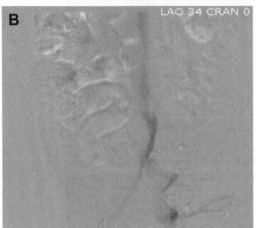

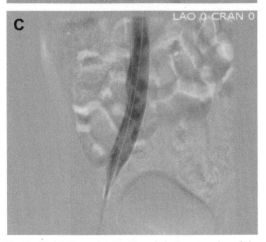

Fig. 9. Right iliac vein stenting. (*A*) Venography of the right external iliac vein demonstrates flattening of the right external iliac vein with subsequent retrograde flow into the right internal iliac vein into pelvic collateral veins (*B*). (*C*) Stenting of the right external into the common iliac vein with bare-metal stent improved antegrade flow in the right iliac venous system.

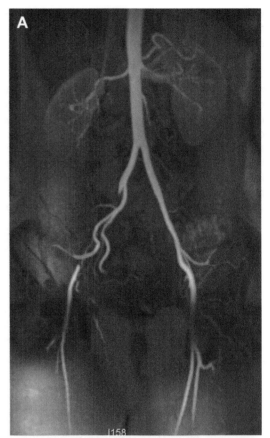

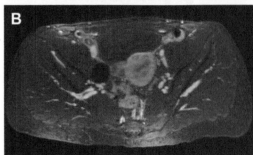

Fig. 10. External iliac artery endofibrosis. (*A*) MIP image from contrast-enhanced MR angiography of a female patient demonstrate a long segment of diffuse severe narrowing in the right external iliac artery. (*B*) Axial images demonstrate thickening of the arterial wall of the right external iliac artery compatible with fibrosis of the intimal wall, endofibrosis.

pelvic MR venogram demonstrated greater than 50% extrinsic compression of the right common and external iliac veins along with pelvic venous collateralization and reversal of flow in the right internal iliac vein (see **Fig.** 8B–E). Based on the MR finding, the patient was taken for venography and IVUS evaluation of the right iliac vein, which confirmed right iliac vein compression with associated reversal of flow in the right internal iliac vein with pelvic vein collateralization (**Fig.** 9A, B). The right iliac vein was stented and poststenting images demonstrated improved flow in the right iliac vein (see **Fig.** 9C).

A few reports have described external iliac vein thrombosis in avid cyclists previously.[46,47] Much more literature is available on the arterial complications from cycling, including external iliac artery endofibrosis and stenosis.[48–50] External iliac artery endofibrosis associated with cycling is typically observed in high-end endurance competitive

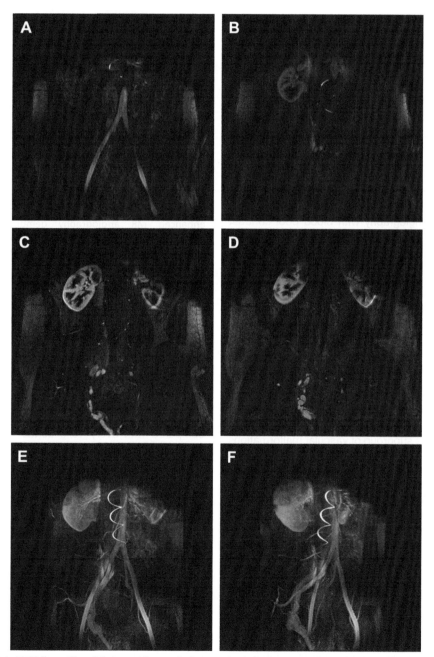

Fig. 11. Pelvic AVM found in a 28-year-old man during work-up for cryptogenic stroke. (*A–D*) Multiple sequential fat-suppressed gadofosveset-enhanced images in the coronal plane shown anterior to posterior reveal a right internal iliac artery to right internal iliac vein pelvic AVM. (*E, F*) MIP images from gadofosveset-enhanced MR imaging further demonstrating the pelvic AVM in the anterior posterior and oblique projections.

cyclists but has also been reported in triathletes, runners, and speed skaters. The entity was first described in 1984 and the classical presentation is that the cyclists are asymptomatic at rest but complain of claudication symptoms and loss of power at peak intensity.[51] Angiographically, the segment of endofibrosis in the external iliac artery has been described as a long 5- to 6-cm segment of diffuse narrowing. Right external iliac artery endofibrosis is shown in a female patient in **Fig. 10**. It is has been proposed that the same repetitive microtrauma from cycling believed to cause external iliac artery endofibrosis may also lead to injury and compression of the iliac vein.[46]

Pelvic Arteriovenous Malformations

A 28-year-old man presented with symptoms of stroke. Patient history revealed no risk factors for stroke; thus, work-up for cryptogenic stroke was initiated. Echocardiogram with bubble study revealed a patent foramen ovale but lower extremity ultrasound was negative for femoropopliteal DVT. Pelvic MR angiography with blood pool contrast agent was then performed to evaluate for occult pelvic DVT and the presence of predisposing factor for DVT, such as left common iliac vein compression. No signs of iliac vein compression were identified, and, unexpectedly, a pelvic arteriovenous malformation (AVM) in the right pelvis was identified (**Fig. 11**). Arterial-phase images obtained in the coronal plane are shown in **Fig. 11A–D** in an anterior to posterior progression to demonstrate the hypertrophied tortuous right internal iliac artery. MIPs are shown in **Fig. 11E–F** in 2 different projections to demonstrate the feeding right internal iliac artery as well as the early venous drainage consistent with AVM.

AVMs are a subgroup of vascular malformations characterized by high blood flow. Unlike AVFs (**Fig. 12**), which are a direct connection between a single artery and a single vein without an intervening capillary bed, AVMs are complex lesions with a nidus of dysplastic vascular channels that connect feeding arteries to draining veins.[52] The absence of a capillary bed between the arteries and veins leads to high flow with low resistance. In some cases, this low-resistance flow can lead to high-output congestive heart failure.[53] AVMs are present at birth but often do not become evident clinically until childhood or adulthood, particularly if an AVM is located in a deep structure, such as the pelvis. Pelvic AVMs are especially rare in men with the majority of AVM distributed in the extremities or neck and face.[53]

In this case, the pelvic AVM discovered incidentally in the work-up of cryptogenic stroke in the

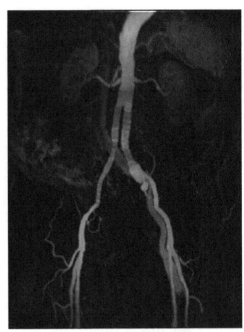

Fig. 12. AV fistula. MIP image from contrast-enhanced MR angiography demonstrates early contrast filling of the left femoral vein consistent with a left-sided femoral artery to left femoral vein AVF.

aforementioned 28-year-old man. The dynamic contrast-enhanced sequences with gadofosveset were helpful in identifying and characterizing the pelvic AVM. If the AVM had been suspected prior to the MR, further characterization could have been performed with 3-D dynamic time-resolved MR angiography. The main advantage of dynamic time-resolved MR angiography is that it allows the acquisition of a 3-D data set every 2 seconds compared with every 15 seconds with conventional acquisition sequences. This increased temporal resolution allows for the precise characterization between low and high flow vascular malformations as well as direction of blood flow and characterization between the arteries and veins.[52]

Priapism

An occasional indication for pelvic MR angiography is for the evaluation of priapism. Priapism refers to prolonged erection (>4 hours) in the absence of sexual activity or other physical or psychological stimulation. It is considered a urologic emergency and failure to adequately treat priapism can lead to diminished sexual function, impotence, and in severe cases penile necrosis.[54] Priapism is divided into 2 categories: nonischemic (high flow) and ischemic (low flow). The vast

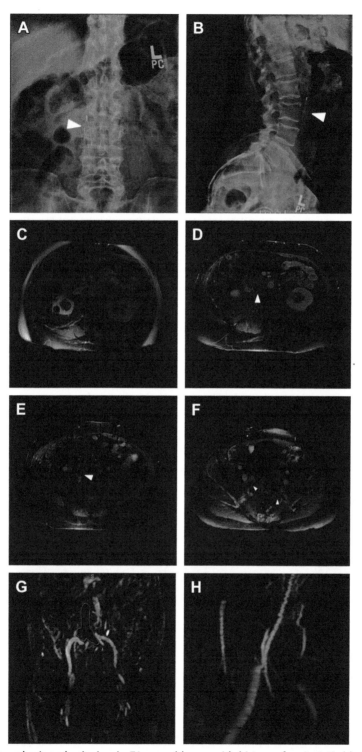

Fig. 13. Iliocaval thrombosis and priapism in 71-year-old man with history of metastatic bladder cancer. (*A, B*) Frontal and lateral radiographs reveal the presence of an IVC filter (*arrowheads*). (*C–F*) Fat-suppressed gadopentetate-enhanced axial images at multiple levels demonstrate thrombus extending from the IVC filter into the bilateral common iliac veins and into the left internal iliac vein (*arrowheads*). (*G*) Coronal image, thrombus has been outlined in red for improved visualization. (*H*) TOF MIP demonstrating no flow in the bilateral common iliac veins and lumbar vein collateralization.

majority of priapism (80%–90%) is ischemic in etiology.[54] There are several potential causes of ischemic priapism including, but not limited to, neurologic, malignant, sickle-cell disease, thrombotic, related to adverse effects from medications, or illicit drugs.[55]

Nonischemic priapism was first described in the literature in 1960 in a man who developed arteriosinusoidal fistulas and nonischemic priapism after traumatic injury sustained during coitus.[56] The arteriosinusoidal fistulas in high-flow nonischemic priapism allow for increased low-resistance inflow to the penis, resulting in priapism. As the category implies, nonischemic priapism results in the delivery of oxygenated blood to the penis and does not require immediate intervention because there is no risk of tissue loss. In addition, the penis is not typically painful and the penis is nonrigid.[55]

Initial diagnostic imaging evaluation of priapism is usually performed with penile Doppler ultrasound. Both nonischemic and ischemic priapism have distinct Doppler ultrasound characteristics that enable a rapid distinction. The pattern of arterial inflow on ultrasound evaluation in nonischemic priapism is normal or increased peak systolic velocity in the cavernosal arteries with low resistive indices indicating low-resistance flow. Additionally, high flow may be observed in an engorged dorsal vein compatible with the high ingress and egress of blood from the penis characteristic of high-flow priapism. Conversely, Doppler ultrasound of ischemic priapism reveals low or absent velocity with high-resistance to flow and flow in the dorsal vein is either absent or poor. Sinusoidal thrombosis may also be evident on ultrasound.

Further evaluation of nonischemic priapism is usually performed with angiography to identify and characterize the AVF. Treatment is with transcatheter embolization of the cavernosal artery, a terminal branch of the pudendal and penile arteries. Ischemic priapism, in contrast, requires emergent aspiration of cavernosal blood to prevent thrombosis and fibrosis and the associated sequelae of erectile dysfunction.

A 71-year-old man with history of metastatic transitional cell carcinoma of the bladder with history of DVT and pulmonary embolus status post-IVC filter placement (**Fig. 13**A, B) 6 months prior developed acute onset of positional priapism. Examination revealed a turgid penis in the standing position, which was relieved in either the supine or sitting position. The patient was referred for MR angiography to differentiate between metastatic disease or thrombus as the mechanism of obstruction of venous outflow. Gadolinium-enhanced MR angiography demonstrated a filling

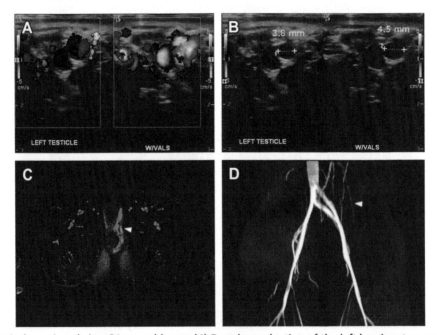

Fig. 14. Testicular varicocele in a 31-year-old man. (*A*) Doppler evaluation of the left hemiscrotum reveals multiple dilated tortuous vessels. (*B*) The dilated veins of the pampiniform plexus measure 3.8 mm and increase to 4.5 mm with the Valsalva maneuver. (*C*) Fat-suppressed gadofosveset-enhanced images demonstrate pooling of contrast in dilated veins (*arrowhead*) in the left hemiscrotum. (*D*) TOF images demonstrate a duplicated left common iliac vein, a rare incidental finding. The left spermatic vein is denoted by the arrowhead. The left spermatic vein is poorly visualized peripherally suggesting slow flow or reversal of flow.

defect extending from the IVC filter into the iliac veins bilaterally and into the left internal iliac vein on the left (see **Fig. 13C–G**). TOF MIP images demonstrate absence of signal in the common iliac veins bilaterally with extensive lumbar collateralization (see **Fig. 13H**). Coumadin (warfarin) was initiated and the patient's positional priapism resolved within 2 weeks.

Testicular Varicocele

Testicular varicocele refers to the dilation of the veins of the pampiniform plexus and has been associated with scrotal swelling, heaviness, pressure, pain, and fatigue. In addition, diminished fertility has been described as a complication of testicular varicocele.[57] Varicoceles are seen in approximately 15% of the male population.[58,59] The mechanism of varicocele development remains unclear but given the increased frequency of left-sided to right-sided varicoceles, an approximately 10-to-1 ratio, many investigators have attributed this increased frequency to the perpendicular insertion of the left spermatic vein into the left renal vein.[60] The right spermatic vein, in contrast, has an oblique insertion into the IVC. Isolated right testicular varicocele is rare and, when encountered, merits additional evaluation to exclude extrinsic compression of the right spermatic vein, such as from mass lesion.

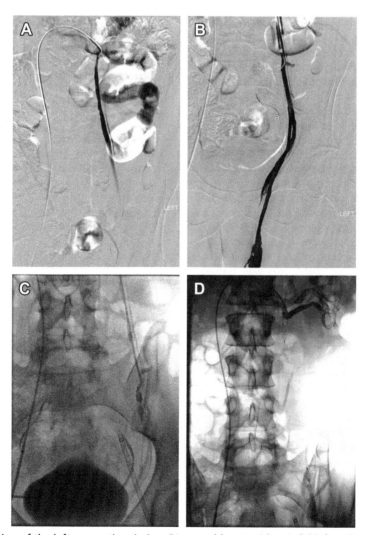

Fig. 15. Embolization of the left spermatic vein in a 31-year-old man with painful left varicocele. (*A, B*) Venography of the left spermatic vein via the left renal vein demonstrates retrograde flow in the left spermatic vein to the level of the left hemiscrotum. (*C*) An Amplatzer Plug 4 is placed in the distal left spermatic vein. (*D*) Post-embolization venography after placement of a second Amplatzer plug in the proximal left spermatic vein demonstrates occlusion of the left spermatic vein.

Physical examination and ultrasound evaluation are important in the initial evaluation and characterization of testicular varicocele. On ultrasound evaluation, the varicocele may appear as anechoic tubular structures that demonstrate flow on Doppler evaluation. More than 2 veins of the pampiniform plexus should be visualized. Dilated vessels greater than 3 mm that expand in size with the Valsalva maneuver are suggestive of varicocele; other investigators have reported using a threshold of greater than 2 mm.[59] Patients should be evaluated in both supine and standing positions. Ultrasound has a high sensitivity for the detection of varicocele (93%) versus 71% for physical examination when compared with venography as the gold standard.[61] MR angiography can be further used to evaluate for preoperative planning either through a surgical or endovascular approach.

A 31-year-old man presented with symptoms of left-sided scrotal swelling, heaviness, and achiness of his scrotum. The patient described worsening discomfort with weight lifting. Physical examination revealed enlargement of the left hemiscrotum with palpation similar to a bag of worms. In comparison with the right testicle, the left testicle was smaller in size. Ultrasound evaluation demonstrated multiple dilated tortuous veins of the pampiniform plexus, which increased from 3.8 mm to 4.5 mm with the Valsalva maneuver (**Fig. 14**A, B). MR imaging, similarly, revealed dilated and tortuous left spermatic vein to the level of the testicle compatible with varicocele identified on both physical examination and ultrasound (see **Fig. 14**C). The left spermatic vein was partially imaged on TOF images, suggesting the possibility of retrograde flow in the spermatic vein. A duplicated left common iliac vein was also incidentally found (see **Fig. 14**D). No mass lesions or extrinsic compression of the left spermatic vein was identified on MR imaging.

The patient was then taken for endovascular treatment of the left-sided varicocele given his significant discomfort, which was interfering with the quality of his life. Left spermatic vein venography demonstrated reversal of flow of the left spermatic vein, as suggested on ultrasound and MR (**Fig. 15**A, B), with reversal of flow to the level of the dilated pampiniform plexus at the level of the testicle. An Amplatzer Vascular Plug 4 was deployed in the distal left spermatic vein (see **Fig. 15**C). Left spermatic vein venography after the placement of a second Amplatzer Vascular Plug 4 (St. Jude Medical, St. Paul, MN, USA) in the proximal left spermatic vein demonstrated successful occlusion of the left spermatic vein (see **Fig. 15**D).

SUMMARY

MR angiography is a powerful tool in evaluating anatomy and pathology when applied to the male pelvis. MR angiography produces high-quality images of the arterial system approaching the resolution of CT angiography, without ionizing radiation. Additional advantages include the ability to obtain angiographic images in the absence of contrast material with non–contrast-enhanced MR angiographic techniques, which may be necessary in patients with renal disease or with allergy. The recent introduction of blood pool contrast agents, such as gadofosveset, has significantly improved the quality of imaging of the venous system, because it is no longer dependent on the first-pass imaging. Steady state imaging with blood pool contrast agents allows for the acquisition of superior-quality high-resolution images and other time-intensive techniques. The extended imaging time also allows for the testing for functional consequences of provocative maneuvers.

REFERENCES

1. Schneider G. Magnetic resonance angiography techniques, indications, and practical applications. New York: Springer; 2005. Available at: <http://public.eblib.com/EBLPublic/PublicView.do?ptiID=304829>.
2. Neri E, Cosottini M, Caramella D. MR angiography of the body: techniques and clinical applications. London: Springer; 2011.
3. Goyen M. Gadofosveset-enhanced magnetic resonance angiography. Vasc Health Risk Manag 2008; 4:1–9.
4. Sabach AS, Bruno M, Kim D, et al. Gadofosveset trisodium: abdominal and peripheral vascular applications. Am J Roentgenol 2013;200:1378–86.
5. Shamsi K, Yucel EK, Chamberlin P. A summary of safety of gadofosveset (MS-325) at 0.03 mmol/kg body weight dose: phase II and Phase III clinical trials data. Invest Radiol 2006;41:822–30.
6. Rohrer M, Bauer H, Mintorovitch J, et al. Comparison of magnetic properties of MRI contrast media solutions at different magnetic field strengths. Invest Radiol 2005;40:715–24.
7. Aime S, Caravan P. Biodistribution of gadolinium-based contrast agents, including gadolinium deposition. J Magn Reson Imaging 2009;30:1259–67.
8. Bremerich J, Bilecen D, Reimer P. MR angiography with blood pool contrast agents. Eur Radiol 2007; 17:3017–24.
9. Weissleder R, Elizondo G, Wittenberg J, et al. Ultrasmall superparamagnetic iron oxide: characterization of a new class of contrast agents for MR imaging. Radiology 1990;175:489–93.

10. Weissleder R, Elizondo G, Wittenberg J, et al. Ultra-small superparamagnetic iron oxide: an intravenous contrast agent for assessing lymph nodes with MR imaging. Radiology 1990;175:494–8.

11. Harisinghani MG, Barentsz J, Hahn PF, et al. Noninvasive detection of clinically occult lymph-node metastases in prostate cancer. N Engl J Med 2003;348:2491–9.

12. Harisinghani MG, Dixon WT, Saksena MA, et al. MR Lymphangiography: imaging Strategies to Optimize the Imaging of Lymph Nodes with Ferumoxtran-10. Radiographics 2004;24:867–78.

13. Lu M, Cohen MH, Rieves D, et al. FDA report: Ferumoxytol for intravenous iron therapy in adult patients with chronic kidney disease. Am J Hematol 2010;85:315–9.

14. Li W, Tutton S, Vu AT, et al. First-pass contrast-enhanced magnetic resonance angiography in humans using ferumoxytol, a novel ultrasmall superparamagnetic iron oxide (USPIO)-based blood pool agent. J Magn Reson Imaging 2005;21:46–52.

15. Sigovan M, Gasper W, Alley HF, et al. USPIO-enhanced MR angiography of arteriovenous fistulas in patients with renal failure. Radiology 2012;265:584–90.

16. Horejs D, Gilbert PM, Burstein S, et al. Normal aortoiliac diameters by CT. J Comput Assist Tomogr 1988;12:602–3.

17. Moore KL. Before we are born: essentials of embryology and birth defects. Philadelphia: Saunders/Elsevier; 2013.

18. Fătu C, Puişoru M, Fătu IC. Morphometry of the internal iliac artery in different ethnic groups. Ann Anat 2006;188:541–6.

19. Yamaki K, Saga T, Doi Y, et al. A statistical study of the branching of the human internal iliac artery. Kurume Med J 1998;45:333–40.

20. Bilhim T, Casal D, Furtado A, et al. Branching patterns of the male internal iliac artery: imaging findings. Surg Radiol Anat 2010;33:151–9.

21. Bilhim T, Tinto HR, Fernandes L, et al. Radiological anatomy of prostatic arteries. Tech Vasc Interv Radiol 2012;15:276–85.

22. Awad A, Alsaid B, Bessede T, et al. Evolution in the concept of erection anatomy. Surg Radiol Anat 2011;33:301–12.

23. Pereira JA, Bilhim T, Rio Tinto H, et al. Radiologic anatomy of arteriogenic erectile dysfunction: a systematized approach. Acta Med Port 2013;26:219–25.

24. Smith JC, Gregorius JC, Breazeale BH, et al. The corona mortis, a frequent vascular variant susceptible to blunt pelvic trauma: identification at routine multidetector CT. J Vasc Interv Radiol 2009;20:455–60.

25. Hadizadeh DR, Gieseke J, Lohmaier SH, et al. Peripheral MR angiography with blood pool contrast agent: prospective intraindividual comparative study of high-spatial-resolution steady-state MR angiography versus standard-resolution first-pass MR angiography and DSA. Radiology 2008;249:701–11.

26. Sandhu RS, Pipinos II. Isolated iliac artery aneurysms. Semin Vasc Surg 2005;18:209–15.

27. Johnston KW, Rutherford RB, Tilson MD, et al. Suggested standards for reporting on arterial aneurysms. Subcommittee on Reporting Standards for Arterial Aneurysms, Ad Hoc Committee on Reporting Standards, Society for Vascular Surgery and North American Chapter, International Society for Cardiovascular Surgery. J Vasc Surg 1991;13:452–8.

28. Bacharach JM, Slovut DP. State of the art: management of iliac artery aneurysmal disease. Catheter Cardiovasc Interv 2008;71:708–14.

29. Sakamoto I, Sueyoshi E, Hazama S, et al. Endovascular treatment of iliac artery aneurysms. Radiographics 2005;25(Suppl 1):S213–27.

30. Buckley CJ, Buckley SD. Technical tips for endovascular repair of common iliac artery aneurysms. Semin Vasc Surg 2008;21:31–4.

31. Uberoi R, Tsetis D, Shrivastava V, et al. Standard of practice for the interventional management of isolated iliac artery aneurysms. Cardiovasc Intervent Radiol 2010;34:3–13.

32. Schoenwolf GC, Bleyl SB, Brauer PR, et al. Larsen's human embryology. 4th edition. Philadelphia: Churchill Livingstone/Elsevier; 2009.

33. Lewis M, Yanny S, Malcolm PN. Advantages of blood pool contrast agents in MR angiography: a pictorial review. J Med Imaging Radiat Oncol 2012;56:187–91.

34. Safavi-Abbasi S, Reis C, Talley MC, et al. Rudolf Ludwig Karl Virchow: pathologist, physician, anthropologist, and politician. Implications of his work for the understanding of cerebrovascular pathology and stroke. Neurosurg Focus 2006;20:E1.

35. May R, Thurner J. The cause of the predominantly sinistral occurrence of thrombosis of the pelvic veins. Angiology 1957;8:419–27.

36. Ahmed HK, Hagspiel KD. Intravascular ultrasonographic findings in May-Thurner syndrome (iliac vein compression syndrome). J Ultrasound Med 2001;20:251–6.

37. Brazeau NF, Harvey HB, Pinto EG, et al. May-Thurner syndrome: diagnosis and management. VASA 2013;42(2):96–105.

38. Gurel K, Gurel S, Karavas E, et al. Direct contrast-enhanced MR venography in the diagnosis of May-Thurner syndrome. Eur J Radiol 2011;80:533–6.

39. Kalu S, Shah P, Natarajan A, et al. May-thurner syndrome: a case report and review of the literature. Case Rep Vasc Med 2013;2013:740182.

40. Raju S, Neglen P. High prevalence of nonthrombotic iliac vein lesions in chronic venous disease: a permissive role in pathogenicity. J Vasc Surg 2006;44:136–43 [discussion: 144].

41. Kibbe MR, Ujiki M, Goodwin AL, et al. Iliac vein compression in an asymptomatic patient population. J Vasc Surg 2004;39:937–43.

42. McDermott S, Oliveira G, Ergul E, et al. May-thurner syndrome: can it be diagnosed on a single magnetic resonance venography study? Diagn Interv Radiol 2012. http://dx.doi.org/10.4261/1305-3825.DIR.5939-12.1.

43. Canales JF, Krajcer Z. Intravascular ultrasound guidance in treating May-Thurner syndrome. Tex Heart Inst J 2010;37:496–7.

44. O'Sullivan GJ, Semba CP, Bittner CA, et al. Endovascular management of iliac vein compression (May-Thurner) syndrome. J Vasc Interv Radiol 2000;11:823–36.

45. Patel NH, Stookey KR, Ketcham DB, et al. Endovascular management of acute extensive iliofemoral deep venous thrombosis caused by May-Thurner syndrome. J Vasc Interv Radiol 2000;11:1297–302.

46. Salam A, Chung J, Milner R. External iliac vein stenosis owing to prolonged cycling. Vascular 2010;18:111–5.

47. Nakamura KM, Skeik N, Shepherd RF, et al. External iliac vein thrombosis in an athletic cyclist with a history of external iliac artery endofibrosis and thrombosis. Vasc Endovascular Surg 2012;45:761–4.

48. Chevalier JM, Enon B, Walder J, et al. Endofibrosis of the external iliac artery in bicycle racers: an unrecognized pathological state. Ann Vasc Surg 1986;1:297–303.

49. Falor AE, Zobel M, De Virgilio C. External iliac artery fibrosis in endurance athletes successfully treated with bypass grafting. Ann Vasc Surg 2013. http://dx.doi.org/10.1016/j.avsg.2013.01.012.

50. Shalhub S, Zierler RE, Smith W, et al. Vasospasm as a cause for claudication in athletes with external iliac artery endofibrosis. J Vasc Surg 2013;58:105–11.

51. Walder J, Mosimann F, Van Melle G, et al. Iliac endofibrosis in 2 cycling racers. Helv Chir Acta 1985;51:793–5 [in French].

52. Flors L, Leiva-Salinas C, Maged IM, et al. MR imaging of soft-tissue vascular malformations: diagnosis, classification, and therapy follow-up. Radiographics 2011;31:1321–40 [discussion: 1340–1].

53. Tanaka M, Iida K, Matsumoto S, et al. A case of pelvic arteriovenous malformation in a male. Int J Urol 1999;6:374–6.

54. Alhalbouni S, Deem S, Abu-Halimah S, et al. Atypical presentation of priapism in a patient with acute iliocaval deep venous thrombosis secondary to may-thurner syndrome. Vasc Endovascular Surg 2013;47:488–92.

55. Halls JE, Patel DV, Walkden M, et al. Priapism: pathophysiology and the role of the radiologist. Br J Radiol 2012;85(Spec No 1):S79–85.

56. Burt FB, Schirmer HK, Scott WW. A new concept in the management of priapism. J Urol 1960;83:60–1.

57. Iaccarino V, Venetucci P. Interventional radiology of male varicocele: current status. Cardiovasc Intervent Radiol 2012;35:1263–80.

58. Meacham RB, Townsend RR, Rademacher D, et al. The incidence of varicoceles in the general population when evaluated by physical examination, gray scale sonography and color Doppler sonography. J Urol 1994;151:1535–8.

59. Beddy P, Geoghegan T, Browne RF, et al. Testicular varicoceles. Clin Radiol 2005;60:1248–55.

60. Fretz PC, Sandlow JI. Varicocele: current concepts in pathophysiology, diagnosis, and treatment. Urol Clin North Am 2002;29:921–37.

61. Petros JA, Andriole GL, Middleton WD, et al. Correlation of testicular color Doppler ultrasonography, physical examination and venography in the detection of left varicoceles in men with infertility. J Urol 1991;145:785–8.

Index

Note: Page numbers of article titles are in **boldface** type.

A

Aneurysm(s), of iliac artery, endovascular repair
　　of, 245
　　　　fat-suppressed contrast-enhanced coronal
　　　　　　images of, 245
Artemis fusion device, 138, 141
Arterial system, pelvic, anatomy of, 242–243
Arteriovenous malformations, pelvic, 251, 252
Artery, external iliac, 242
　　iliac, aneurysm(s) of, endovascular repair of, 245
　　　　fat-suppressed contrast-enhanced coronal
　　　　　　images of, 245
　　internal iliac, 242–243
Atherosclerotic disease, 244

B

Bladder, anatomy of, 130–131
　　cancer of, biology of, 129–130
　　　　computed tomography in, 129
　　　　etiologic factors in, 129
　　　　imaging of, 151–153
　　　　incidence of, 129
　　　　metastatis to pelvic wall muscle, 210
　　　　MR imaging protocol for, 131–132
　　　　MR imaging staging of, N staging, 133
　　　　　　T staging, 132–133, 134
　　　　staging of, 130, 131, 132
　　carcinoma of, pelvic spread of, 204–205
　　　　tumors metastatic to, 207–208
　　lesions of, imaging pathway for, 131
　　MR imaging of, **129–134**
　　normal, 202
　　squamous cell carcinomas and, 129–130
　　transitional cell carcinoma of, muscle-sparing
　　　　versus muscle-invasive, 151, 152
Bladder wall, flat transitional cell carcinoma of, on
　　diffusion-weighted imaging, 152, 153
Bone, metastatic lesions to, in pelvis, 209–212
Bowel, and rectum, 153–157

C

Colorectal cancer, introduction to, 153
　　mortality associated with, 165
Computed tomography, in bladder cancer, 129
Crohn disease, active, diffusion-weighted
　　imaging of, 157

D

Denonvilliers fascia, 172
Diffusion-weighted imaging, in disease
　　detection, 145
　　in flat transitional cell carcinoma of bladder
　　　　wall, 152, 153
　　in prostate cancer, 148–151
　　in rectal cancer, 168–169
　　in scrotal lesions, 218, 219
　　interpretation of, 146–147
　　limitations of, 147
　　of active Crohn disease, 157
　　of inflammatory bowel disease, 156–157
　　of lymph nodes of male pelvis, 159
　　of male pelvis, **145–163**
　　of prostate, 147–151
　　　　technical considerations in, 147
　　of rectal cancer, 153–156
　　of testes, 157–158
　　technical aspects of, 146
　　technique of, principles of, 145–146
Dynamic contrast-enhanced subtracted MR
　　imaging, in scrotal lesions, 218–219, 227, 228

E

Embryonal carcinoma, of testis, 224, 225
Endofibrosis, of external iliac artery, 250, 252
Epidermoid cysts, testicular, 229, 231
Epididymitis, scrotal, 234
Epididymo-orchitis, 233

G

Gadolinium-based contrast agent, for MR
　　angiography, 240–241
Germ cell tumor, mixed, of testis, 224, 229
Granulomatous orchitis, 230, 232

I

Iliac vein, right, compression of, 249–252
Iliocaval thrombosis, priapism and, 253, 254–255
Inflammatory bowel disease, background of, 156
　　diffusion-weighted imaging of, 156–157
Intratesticular masses, 222–228
　　benign, 228–230

1064-9689/14/$ – see front matter © 2014 Elsevier Inc. All rights reserved.

mri.theclinics.com

Moving?

Make sure your subscription moves with you!

To notify us of your new address, find your **Clinics Account Number** (located on your mailing label above your name), and contact customer service at:

Email: journalscustomerservice-usa@elsevier.com

800-654-2452 (subscribers in the U.S. & Canada)
314-447-8871 (subscribers outside of the U.S. & Canada)

Fax number: 314-447-8029

Elsevier Health Sciences Division
Subscription Customer Service
3251 Riverport Lane
Maryland Heights, MO 63043

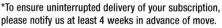
*To ensure uninterrupted delivery of your subscription, please notify us at least 4 weeks in advance of move.

ELSEVIER

Printed and bound by CPI Group (UK) Ltd, Croydon, CR0 4YY

03/10/2024

01040379-0007